Smawcastellane
information services

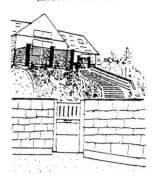

GW00726077

DRUGS, MEDICATIONS
and the EYE

Michael J. Doughty, PhD
Professor

1999
3rd EDITION

E-Mail M.Doughty@gcal.ac.uk
FAX 0141-331-3387
TEL 0141-331-3393

DRUGS, MEDICATIONS and the EYE
CONTENTS 1999

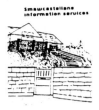

PRINCIPLES OF DRUG ACTION

Purpose of chapter. Any consideration of drug actions requires considerations of the overall mechanism and characteristics of drug effects in the human body; these considerations reflect the pharmacodynamics and pharmacokinetics. The principles of drug receptor theory will thus be presented. Since an understanding of the clinical use of drugs is also important, pharmacokinetic principles and the factors that affect the time-dependent response of the body to drugs will also be covered.

The mechanism(s) underlying drug action is important. For every drug that is legally administered to the human body (for whatever reason and by whatever route), at least some idea of its mechanisms of action is known. These mechanisms both apply to the normal tissues of the body, and especially to the disease or condition for which the drug is being administered (by a health care professional) or being taken (by a patient). Such knowledge of the pharmacodynamics of a drug generally distinguishes a medication (containing drugs) from a chemical being administered to try to manage some bodily ailment or that is causing a toxic reaction.

Pharmacodynamics is a way of describing the molecular action of a drug. Full details of the actual molecular mechanisms of a drug may however not be known, and such details are not always required in order for a drug to be licenced for human use. Thus for newer classes of drugs approved for clinical use, significant controversy may exist concerning actual mechanisms. However, the overall principles for defining the pharmacodynamics are well established and it is these principles that will be followed in defining how a drug exerts a particular clinical action.

Practitioner-oriented pharmaceutical directories for Prescription-Only-Medicines (**PoM**'s) [e.g. MIMS or the BNF- see Chapter 19] often contain a section called the "pharmacology" of a drug. This pharmacological profile may include details of the mode of administration (the *pharmaceutics*), the time base and magnitude of drug action after administration (the *pharmacokinetics*) and the mechanism of action of the drug (the *pharmacodynamics*).

1. PRINCIPLES OF RECEPTOR THEORY (PHARMACODYNAMICS).

When a drug is administered to the body, it will end up at discrete sites within the body, i.e. the sites of action. In cellular and molecular terms, the sites of action are called "receptors". These receptors have several types -

(i) proteinaceous receptors that are present on cells in a tissue, and are identified by what are termed drug binding studies. A drug may bind to such proteinaceous receptors (and "activate" or "block" it), or may bind and modify the action of a natural neurotransmitter or other biological molecule on that receptor; the modification may mimic the neurotransmitter action or to block the action of the neurotransmitter.

(ii) an <u>enzymes as receptors</u>. Enzyme activities are present in the fluids of the body, on the surface of cells, or inside cells. Drugs can bind to the enzyme, and may inhibit or increase its activity. The change in activity may indirectly change the levels of neurotransmitters or other molecules.

(iii) a <u>cell membrane</u>. Some drugs are characterized only by their ability to generally alter membrane functions of cells and, as a result, can prevent the normal electrophysiological activity of that membrane or generally perturb the function of the membrane in controlling the integrity of the cell.

EXAMPLES for STUDY

(i))(a) phenylephrine (e.g. as found in PoM **Minims**[R] **Phenylephrine Hydrochloride** eye-drops) is a drug that binds to *alpha*$_1$-adrenergic proteinaceous receptor molecules that are present on the iris dilator muscle. As a result of this binding, the phenylephrine causes the smooth muscle of the dilator to contract. Since epinephrine (adrenaline) will also produce the same contraction, the phenylephrine mimics the action of epinephrine and so can be referred to as a sympathomimetic, specifically an *alpha*$_1$-adrenoceptor stimulant.

(i)(b) **salbutamol** (e.g. as found in PoM **Ventolin**[R] tablets) is a drug that binds to *beta*$_2$-adrenergic proteinaceous receptors in the smooth muscles of the tracheobronchial lining. As a result of the binding, the salbutamol causes these muscles to relax and more air can be taken in with an intake of breath. Since epinephrine (adrenaline) can produce the same relaxation, the salbutamol is also a sympathomimetic but a *beta*$_2$-adrenoceptor stimulant.

(i)(c) metoprolol (e.g. as found in PoM **Lopresor**[R] tablets) binds to *beta*$_1$- and *beta*$_2$-adrenoceptors on the heart and tracheobronchial tissue. As a result of the binding to the heart tissue, the heart rate is slowed and, as a result of binding to the tracheobronchial smooth muscles, these muscles contract (and close down the airways). Since these actions are opposite to adrenaline, metoprolol is classified as a *beta*-adrenoceptor blocker.

(ii)(a) donepezil (e.g. as found in PoM **Aricept**[R] tablets) is a drug that binds to the enzyme acetylcholinesterase and inhibits it; the drug is thus an anti-cholinesterase. Since this enzyme normally breaks down the neurotransmitter acetylcholine, the inhibition results in elevation in the levels of acetylcholine. The donepezil thus produces acetylcholine-like effects and so is a parasympathomimetic drug. Since the drug does not directly change the action of acetylcholine on its receptor, it is an indirect-acting parasympathomimetic.

(ii)(b) dorzolamide (e.g. as found in PoM **Trusopt**[R] eye drops) binds to an enzyme in the tissues and plasma called carbonic anhydrase and inhibits the enzyme activity; acetazolamide is thus a carbonic anhydrase (CAI) inhibitor. As a result of the inhibition of CAI, the rates of inter-conversion between CO_2 and bicarbonate are reduced and various types of fluid secretion (including at the ciliary epithelium) are reduced.

(iii) (a) amethocaine (also known as tetracaine) (e.g. as found in PoM **Minims**[R] **Amethocaine Hydrochloride** eye-drops) binds to nerve cell membranes to block nerve conduction. A specific "receptor" for eye tissues has not been identified but anaesthetic drug binding to nerves has some receptor-like properties. Amethocaine produces a topical anaesthetic effects, but can bind non-specifically to other cell membranes.

(iii)(b) polymyxin B sulphate (e.g. as found in PoM **Polyfax**[R] eye ointment) associates with bacterial cell membranes. A specific receptor has not been identified but, as a result of the non-specific binding, the membrane function is greatly perturbed and the bacterium fails to thrive or even dies if high enough drug concentrations are applied.

2. DETERMINATION OF DRUG BINDING or INTERACTION.

The principles of pharmacodynamics are based on the observation that any drug action can be defined by its concentration-dependent effects when mixed with a "receptor" (or presented to the receptor in the living body). Thus there is a concentration when the drug shows just a small ability to bind to the "receptor" (and produce a threshold activation or inhibition), a concentration where many of the "receptors" will easily bind the drug and a concentration at which all of the drug "receptors" have bound the drug (a plateau or saturation effect). All three concentration ranges can be measured in what are called drug binding studies which allow one to define the percent (%) of the receptors that have bound the drug, e.g. 10 %, 50 % or 100 %.

That concentration range where many of the receptors have bound the drug has great medicinal relevance and is usually equated with the 50 % receptor binding. From a molecular perspective, this 50 % drug binding is called the K_d and is a quantitative measure of the affinity of the drug for the receptor. In clinical terms, the drug quantity that needs to be administered is that which essentially produces a 50 % binding and thus a 50 % activity effect; this concentration / quantity is thus known as the ED_{50} [ee-dee-fifty].

The drug can either simply bind to the receptor (a direct binding) and produce an effect, or can bind to a site on the receptor such that it either allows another drug to bind more readily or results in the displacement of another drug. The drug concentration that produces a 50 %change in binding of a second drug can be determined; the latter 50 % effect is usually inhibitory and is called an inhibitory 50 % or I_{50} (eye-fifty).

If the "receptor" is an enzyme, actual drug binding studies are not usually necessary since the actual enzyme activity can be measured instead. However, a drug concentration can be found that produces 10%, 50 % and 100 % inhibition of the activity and thus an I_{50} can be determined.

If the drug interacts with a membrane, the concentration-effect relationships are not so well defined. For nerve membranes, a drug concentration that produces a threshold (minimal) effect can be measured from electrophysiological measurements, or a concentration determined where there is a saturating effect on the nerve membranes. In the first case, just detectable anaesthesia would be produced and in the second case a total loss of sensation (or nerve block) would be achieved. For bacterial membranes, a minimal concentration altering the viability of the microorganisms can be determined; the MIC (or minimum inhibitory concentration).

3. MODELS OF RECEPTORS for ACTIONS OF DRUGS.

In most cases of drug action in the body, the action is via a specific "receptor". Such receptors and the way in which drugs interact with them can be likened to a model of a lock (the receptor) and key (drug). Such physical models allow one to visualise drug actions providing one remembers that such ideas apply to ALL sites of action, i.e. from metoprolol receptors in cardiac membranes, to acetazolamide binding to carbonic anhydrase, to the drug-binding membrane domains for polymyxin B. Sometimes a drug will need to be transported into a cell before it works because the receptors are inside a cell, e.g. most hormone receptors are on the nucleus membrane, and some antibiotics bind to cell ribosomes.

4. DRUG AFFINITY AND POTENCY versus EFFICACY.

There are many practical and clinical consequences of the pharmacodynamic theory of drug action. Since there will usually be a defined range of concentrations over which the drug receptor or target site will operate under the influence of that drug, this concentration range determines the drug quantity (=dose) given to a patient. Since the drug is usually able to "recognise" its receptor (the lock-and-key analogy) only when it is in the vicinity of the receptor over a certain concentration range, the drug has a unique affinity for its receptor. If the concentration of the drug over which this recognition occurs is very low, the drug is a potent one, and *vice versa*. If two drugs that can act on the same receptor are presented simultaneously to the receptor, the more potent (or high affinity) drug will generally displace the less potent (or weak affinity) drug. This applies regardless of whether the drugs "activate" or "block" the receptor.

Clinically, one rarely refers to the potency of a drug simply because so many additional factors determine the action of a drug beyond it being able to bind to a receptor. Thus, in clinical terms, the term efficacy is used as a descriptor for the magnitude of drug effects; a potent drug will generally show a high or substantial efficacy and *vice versa* (but this does not mean that a potent drug has to display high efficacy).

5. DRUG AFFINITY and SELECTIVITY.

Most drug actions at sites in the human body are the result of their interacting with receptors over a discrete concentration range. Some drugs have similarities in molecular structure and will bind to a particular receptor over different discrete concentration ranges, depending on their affinity for that receptor. Drugs that have a very different molecular structure will not bind, but drugs with a similar molecular structure may bind. Drug action can thus be selective, based both on concentration and molecular structure.

EXAMPLES for STUDY of DRUG SELECTIVITY.

Epinephrine (adrenaline) will bind to all adrenergic (adrenaline-binding) receptors, i.e. is non-selective. Phenylephrine will only bind to *alpha*$_1$-adrenergic receptors but not to *beta*-adrenergic receptors. Salbutamol will bind selectively to *beta*$_2$-adrenergic receptors and not to *alpha*-adrenoceptors. Metoprolol will preferentially bind to *beta*$_1$-adrenoceptors, but will show some binding (at high concentrations) to *beta*$_2$-adrenoceptors, although it will not bind to *alpha*-adrenoceptors. Similarly, donepezil binds to acetylcholinesterase (AChE) but not carbonic anhydrase (CA), while dorzolamide binds to CA and not to AcChE.

6. AGONISTS versus ANTAGONISTS.

Drug action on receptors will ordinarily be directional in the sense that the drug either "activates" or "blocks" the receptor site(s). The drug interaction with a receptor can thus produce a positive or agonist effect (in that the activity mediated via that receptor site is augmented), or the drug interaction can produce a negative or antagonist effect (in that the activity mediated via that receptor is attenuated). Agonist drugs can also be called mimetics or stimulants; antagonist drugs can be referred to as lytics or blocking drugs.

Agonists and antagonists can be used in various ways. For example, acetylcholine applied to an iris muscle preparation will cause it to contract; if an ocular drug similar to donepezil (i.e. echothiophate) was also present, then the concentration of acetylcholine required to contract the muscle will be much less because the acetylcholine breakdown is inhibited by the echothiophate acting as an indirect agonist. Alternatively, some agonist drug effects can be counteracted by an antagonist (and *vice versa*). For example, the administration of epinephrine (adrenaline) will open up the airways, increase the pulse and raise blood pressure; metoprolol can block the effects of adrenaline on the pulse and blood pressure at low concentrations but high concentrations are needed to counter the airway effects. A patient with bronchoconstriction (contraction) produced by metoprolol administration (the antagonist) can be helped to breathe by administration of agonists such as epinephrine or salbutamol.

7. TIME BASE OF DRUG ACTION ON RECEPTORS (PHARMACOKINETICS).

For most clinically used drugs, physiological functions are changed as a result of the drug binding to a receptor. However, in most cases, the drug binding is not permanent but temporary. In addition, since the drug-receptor interaction is very much determined by the actual concentration of the drug in the vicinity of the receptors, there are distinct time-dependent changes in the activity (functions) of the receptor as the drug concentration changes in the vicinity of the receptor. That these concentrations will change is determined by the rates of drug movement (delivery) to the sites where the receptors are present and by the rates of drug movement away (wash-out or elimination) from the sites of the receptors. In the simplest sense, one can consider that the blood flow initially carries a drug to a receptor site and then, just as fast, carries the drug away to other parts of the body where there are different receptors. The description of this whole process of drug delivery, absorption and wash-out is called <u>pharmacokinetics</u> and involves the actual measurements of the concentrations of a drug in different parts of the body as a function of the time after the drug was administered. Alternatively, the pharmacokinetics can be indirectly assessed by measuring the time-dependent change in a physiological function (e.g. heart rate); in this case, the term <u>clinical pharmacokinetics</u> is preferable.

The pharmacokinetics of a drug (in a medication) is determined by -

(a) the <u>mode of administration</u> of the drug in the medication, i.e. the pharmaceutical type.

 (b) <u>dose</u>, i.e. the actual quantity (dose) of drug administered.

(c) <u>absorption</u>, i.e. the amount of the drug that is actually absorbed into the body; *bioavailability* is the term for the amount of this absorbed drug.

(d) <u>distribution</u>, i.e. the way in which the drug is distributed throughout the body after being administered. Since the drug in a tablet (for example) will often be distributed throughout the body, its concentration at any one site in the body will be diluted from that in the original pharmaceutical. The term *volume of distribution* is thus used to describe this dilution.

 (e) <u>metabolism</u>. Most drugs are active only until they are broken down by enzymes in the body. This is called *biotransformation*.

 (f) <u>elimination</u> (excretion). Drugs generally do not stay in the body but are usually rapidly eliminated. The route and rate at which the drug is excreted determines the overall pharmacokinetics and the term *bioelimination* is used to describe this.

ALL of these factors have some degree of dependence upon each other. The overall pharmacokinetics of a drug reflect the combined effects of all of these factors and is of great importance in determining the efficacy of pharmaceuticals and whether significant adverse drug reactions (ADR's) will be associated with their use.

EXAMPLES for STUDY of DOSE DEPENDENCE of DRUG ACTIONS.

(a) **phenylephrine** eye-drops. The mode of administration is a solution which is readily compatible with the tear film. A single drop containing 0.12 % w/v phenylephrine should affect the conjunctival vasculature but should not normally affect the pupil. A single drop containing 2.5 % phenylephrine should produce some pupil dilation (mydriasis) but a single drop of a 10 % solution would be expected to produce a greater effect, with both of the higher concentrations producing a massive effect on the conjunctival vasculature. In all cases, some of the phenylephrine will be absorbed into the mucous membranes of the conjunctiva and into the corneal epithelium, but actually most of the dose will be washed down the naso-lacrimal duct and absorbed into the body. The phenylephrine, especially at the higher doses, will also be absorbed into the aqueous humour to be distributed throughout the anterior segment (including the iris tissue) while that drug that enters the naso-lacrimal duct will be distributed throughout the body. The systemically-absorbed and distributed drug can have pronounced systemic effects even though it is diluted by the huge volume of distribution. The phenylephrine, at all sites, will be metabolized by several enzymes (including monoamine oxidase and catechol-O-methyl-transferase) and the phenylephrine will be inactivated. The phenylephrine and its metabolites that are inside the eye will be washed out through the trabecular meshwork into the blood supply to join the drug and metabolites in the blood stream following naso-lacrimal absorption. The drug and its metabolites will be excreted, in the urine primarily.

(b) **metoprolol** tablets. The tablets can contain 10, 20, 40 or 80 mg of drug. A small dose (10 mg) would produce a small anti-hypertensive effect while a large dose (80 mg) would produce a very large anti-hypertensive effect, and even systemic hypotension. The tablet, perhaps taken with water, is swallowed and dissolves in the stomach fluid. Some the drug can then be absorbed, via the intestinal lining and enters the blood stream. If 1/10 th of the drug in the 10 mg tablet actually was absorbed, this 1 mg will then be progressively diluted as the circulation distributes the blood-drug mixture to every part of the body. Some of the drug will act on the vasculature (to produce vasodilatation) and some will act on the heart (to lower the pulse). Some may reach the tracheobronchial system to produce unwanted bronchoconstriction. The effective concentration of the drug, at any designated part of the body at any particular instant in time, will be determined by the extent of this dilution and both the rate of biotransformation and the rate of bioelimination. The drug is biotransformed by enzymes in the liver and is eliminated both in the urine and feces. In addition, some of the drug will actually enter the eye via the ciliary epithelium (and produce a lowering of intra-ocular pressure) and will then be washed out of the body via the aqueous humour, the trabecular meshwork etc.

8. FACTORS AFFECTING PHARMACOKINETICS.

All of these pharmacokinetic parameters can be influenced by secondary factors. The systemic drug delivery will be considered here; ocular pharmacokinetics will be considered in later chapters. These secondary factors are -

(**a**) general health. Effective drug absorption after oral administration requires a healthy stomach and alimentary tract. The volume of distribution is determined by tissue health and good circulation. Biotransformation of many drugs usually requires a healthy liver. Bioelimination often requires a normally functioning alimentary tract and / or kidney.

(**b**) drug-drug interactions (**INT**) are often the cause of adverse drug reactions (**ADR's**) and / or the reason for contraindications (**C/I**) or specific precautions (**S/P**) for use of the drug. One drug may increase or decrease the absorption of another drug (e.g. caffeine is included in some pharmaceuticals to promote absorption of the other ingredients). One drug may change blood pressure and / or blood flow to change the volume of distribution of another drug. One drug could reduce the liver biotransformation of another drug, i.e. making the second drug more effective because it is metabolised less readily so resulting in much higher plasma concentrations over time, e.g. certain chemicals found in processed grapefruit juice have a selective effect on the bioavailability and biotransformation of oral anti-histamines such as terfenadine. Some other drugs (e.g. diuretics) may generally promote urinary output and thus increase the rate of bioelimination of a second drug.

(**c**) presence of other substances, e.g. food, alcohol, illicit drugs etc. To ensure good bioavailability, some drugs must be taken with meals (e.g. oral hypoglycaemic drugs such as chlorpropamide for type II diabetes). Other drugs should not be taken with meals or specific foodstuffs (e.g. tetracycline antibiotics with milk or vegetables). Other drugs should be taken with other substances to reduce irritation (e.g. some anti-arthritis drugs should be taken with a glass of milk). Alcohol or drug abuse can dramatically alter both bioavailability and biotransformation, as well as the volume of distribution and rates of bioelimination of almost any medicinal drug.

(**d**) age, especially the very young versus the very old. Due to either differences in the volume of distribution (very young patients) or the rates of biotransformation (the elderly), drug pharmacokinetics can be very different in patients of different ages.

(**e**) pharmacogenetics. Some individuals metabolise drugs faster or slower than other individuals and this will determine the levels of drugs in the body and how long the drugs stay in the body (e.g. alcohol, the anti-hypertensive drugs such as metoprolol, and anti-tuberculosis drugs such as isoniazid).

(**f**) chronopharmacology. Some drugs can have markedly different effects when administered at different times of the day for day shift versus night shift personnel (e.g. anti-anxiety / tranquilliser drugs such as diazepam).

Since many of these factors can only be found out once a drug is marketed for general use by the population at large, the **Committee on Safety of Medicines** (CSM) requires that any unusual or unexpected response or reaction to a newly-marketed drug (a PoM pharmaceutical) be reported. The initial period of mandatory reporting can last from 6 months to 2 years, depending on how frequently the product is prescribed and / or what its indications for use are. A Yellow Card reporting scheme exists for all health care practitioners, and the same yellow card system is used for reporting ADR's to all other pharmaceuticals (see Chapter 19).

MEDICATIONS or UNDERSTANDING A PATIENT'S MEDICATION LIST AND MAKING OFFICE RECORDS

Purpose of chapter. Any change is normal visual function could be due to age, disease or the medications that a patient is taking. Equally importantly, perhaps the major contraindication to the use of any diagnostic or therapeutic pharmaceutical (i.e. a drug) on a patient is a known allergy or sensitivity to the active ingredients or any other ingredient of the pharmaceutical. One can only know this if an accurate record is obtained of a patient's current medication history and, in some cases, their past medication history. One should also consider whether a patient's concurrent use of other ophthalmic pharmaceuticals or systemic medications could result in an enhanced or reduced response to the pharmaceutical you intend to use, or that they are likely to be prescribed, etc. Last, but not least, a complete medication record for a patient provides an extraordinarily useful insight into the patients actual condition, rather than one having to simply rely on at-the-moment dialogue. It is the goal of this chapter to illustrate the diverse forms of both patient reporting on medications, the diversity of pharmaceutical types used and the reasons for their use.

MEDICATION INFORMATION and HISTORIES

As a practical working guideline, one should NOT expect a patient to volunteer this information. The gathering of the appropriate and correct information on a patient's medications and on the way they are using them is a prerequisite for responsible and safe practice. Medications generally have a brand (proprietary name, usually registered, e.g. PoM **Valium**[R] for the anti-anxiety drug, diazepam). Generic equivalents containing the same drug (diazepam) can also be widely available for many systemic drugs, and some ophthalmic pharmaceuticals. These generics can only carry a non-proprietary name (PoM **Diazepam**), and are often dispensed from hospital pharmacies; a BNF carries some details of generics, but they do change fairly frequently. Some pharmaceuticals are specifically placed on NHS-approved prescription service (designated as ~~NHS~~ **Diazepam**), while the original brand name products are not approved (e.g. NHS Valium). Information on the medications may be presented in several ways -

(**a**) *verbally*. This method may be limited, incomplete, and often in lay language, e.g. heart tablets, water pills, lots of Aspirin[R], etc. In taking this information, it needs to be corrected and it is advisable to check for errors (e.g. by consulting MIMS, or a BNF) before using this information for the patients' records, or for referral letters etc.

(**b**) a *hand-written list*. This is a preferred method to the verbal one. Medications will often be referred to by brand names, but without details of quantities and / or frequency of use. Details of dosing, etc.shoudl be obtained, especially if a patient is symptomatic.

(**c**) a *pharmacy-generated print out*. This type computer print-out will usually have a list of medications as brand names, the type of pharmaceutical and the quantity dispensed, i.e. per tablet, or dose.

Since brand products may change, it is a most useful exercise to translate the brand names into common drug names and enter both on a patients record, e.g. **Lopresor**[R] tablets (metoprolol), 100 mg, *b.d.s* [see next page].

GOALS OF GOOD MEDICATION RECORDS.

A full medication record is a most useful insight into a patient's state of health, state of mind etc. If a patient is symptomatic or showing signs of drug-drug interactions (adverse effects), this information can be used in the diagnosis of their condition as well as make appropriate plans (e.g. referral) for a patient. Some of these goals are to find out -

(a) what medications a patient is taking, or has recently been taking. These medications should preferably be identified by BRAND name, and their main drug(s) ingredients (identified by generic names).

(b) why the patient is taking these medications. This information provides an excellent opportunity to check for accuracy especially in medication use that is communicated verbally.

(c) how much of these medications is a patient taking. The goal here is to get an idea of whether they are taking their medications at a low, medium, or high doses; a MIMS or BNF will provide the normally-used adult dosing.

(d) when are these medications actually being taken. This will assist you in making a diagnosis, especially for symptomatic patients. A drug-drug interaction is more likely during the initial period of medication use.

(e) how long has a patient been taking these medications. This is more important when adverse ocular reactions to drugs are being investigated.

NOTE. It is a very good habit to always check the identify and spelling of medications in a current MIMS (or equivalent). It is also a good approach to medication history to not accept a "medications same as last visit" for patients' records. It is also a very good idea to indicate, on the patients' records, that questions have definitely been asked about medications and allergies, even if the answer to either question is no, e.g. statements such as "no medications reported" should be included in the records.

NOTE. Where there are any uncertainties, concerns or questions about the adequacy and or safety of these medications, a patient can be (and should be) referred back to the physician who prescribed their medications. In some cases, further information can be obtained from pharmaceutical companies.

PRESCRIPTION WRITING

A drugs (i.e. medications) prescription is a document that essentially provides all the information needed for selection and use of a medicine (pharmaceutical). An acceptable prescription contains information on the practitioner, patient name and address, the SUPERSCRIPTION (i.e. the designation for a PoM), product INSCRIPTION (i.e. the BRAND name and strength of the pharmaceutical), SUBSCRIPTION (i.e. volume of bottle to be dispensed, number of tablets etc.), SIGNATURA (abbreviated Sig.) which is the directions for use of the product that is to be given to the patient, details of LABELLING, REFILL INFORMATION and SIGNATURE. A prescription may be refilled a designated number of times, or up to a certain date by a pharmacist.

ABREVIATIONS RELEVANT TO MEDICINES ADMINISTRATION

A number of abbreviations can be legitimately used to describe drug administration to the body. These abbreviations relate to the timing of when medicines are taken and by what route.

Table 1:

TERM	ABREV	TERM	ABREV
once-a-day	*o.d.*	twice-a-day	*b.d.* or *b.d.s.*
3-times-a-day	*t.d.* or *t.d.s.*	4-times-a-day	*q.d.* or *q.d.s.*
in the morning	*o.m.*	at night (before bed)	*o.n.*
as needed	*p.r.n.*	nothing by mouth	*n.b.m.*
before meals	*a.c.*	after meals	*p.c.*
eyedrops	*gtt*	ointment	*ung*
tablets	*tab.* or *tbl.*		
prescription-only medication	PoM	Pharmacy Medicine	P
(general) sales list	(G)SL	controlled drug	CD

DRUG DELIVERY TO THE BODY DRUG and MONITORING

"Drug" information may be communicated by a patient in different ways. Some information is more important and understanding a drug prescription is useful. All this information is of use for a patient's files, and may also be needed by any health care practitioner when a patient's medications record is being communicated to another health care provider. Slang terminology should be avoided if possible when including such information (in any form) in a patient's records or communicating this information to others.

People take or are administered "medications" not "drugs". Medications (i.e. pharmaceuticals) can be administered to the human body by many different methods. Most pharmaceuticals are manufactured and packaged in such a way so as to optimise their actions when administered in a particular mode. This is the recommended method of administration, and all health care practitioners should avoid using pharmaceutical products in a way that was not recommended. The optometric role is to ensure that we understand what patients should be doing with their medications (in terms of the administration of these medications) and be able to answer basic questions on the different modes of administration. These modes of administration are summarised and discussed below -

(a) CONJUNCTIVAL administration. This is the formal term for the route of entry of drugs from an ophthalmic pharmaceutical, across the corneal and conjunctival surfaces, into the eye or the rest of the body.

Ophthalmic pharmaceuticals can be in the form of solutions, suspensions, oils or liquid gels (all of which are instilled into the eye), or can be in the form of ointments or gels (which are applied to the conjunctiva or to the lid margin). Lastly, there are some very special modes which take the form of wafers, inserts, or shields (all of which are touched to, placed upon or inserted into the lower cul-de-sac). Further details of ophthalmic pharmaceuticals are provided in Chapter 3.

(b) NASAL administration. This term describes drug administration across the nasal mucous epithelium and into the peripheral circulation. Many such pharmaceuticals are actually used for local treatment of the nasal mucosa (e.g. nasal decongestants), but the method is also used for systemic drug delivery.

These pharmaceuticals are in the form of fine mists or vapours. The respiratory epithelia are an extension of the nasal mucosa and so the term also applies to pharmaceuticals administered for the bronchial system. These will be used for local therapeutic actions in the upper respiratory and take the form of sprays or as finely dispersed powders that are administered via an inhaler or neubuliser.

(c) BUCCAL / SUBLINGUAL administration. This term describes the administration of drugs across the buccal or lingual epithelia into the peripheral circulation. The pharmaceutical forms are usually lozenges, sprays or vapours.

(d) ORAL administration. Orally-administered pharmaceuticals can enter the body via the buccal epithelia but predominantly are swallowed and then absorbed across the mucosa of the stomach and alimentary (gastro-intestinal) tract.

Oral pharmaceuticals can take the forms of solutions, elixirs (solutions with alcohol), syrups as well as tablets [note ID / BRAND, scoring (PRES-TABS[TM]), colour coating, etc.], capsules, gelcaps, caplets, sustained, extended- or slow-release tablets, sustets etc.

(e) RECTAL administration. The term is used both to imply use of pharmaceuticals for local therapy as well as for specific delivery of drugs, via the lower alimentary (gastro-intestinal) tract mucosal membranes into the peripheral circulation. Rectal pharmaceuticals usually take the form of suppositories, but other insertion devices (including those containing gels) as well as local creams, ointments, gels etc. are available.

(f) VAGINAL administration. Usually for local therapy of the vaginal mucous membrane, and take the form of solutions (douches) or various types of inserts. Vaginal gels can also be used for systemic administration of drugs, again via the peripheral circulation.

(g) EPIDERMAL administration. This term is used for administration of drugs across the dermis and absorption into the peripheral circulation. These pharmaceuticals can be used for local action, or systemic drug delivery. The pharmaceuticals include creams, ointments, gels, powders (including spray on wet or dry sprays) and special transdermal patch delivery systems (that include tapes, filters, pads, patches).

(h) PARENTERAL administration. This term means injection of a pharmaceutical which is a solution. The delivery can be a single dose or continuous (e.g. *i.v.* drip). The injection site can be intravenous (*i.v.*), intramuscular (*i.m.*), subcutaneous (*s.c.*), subconjunctival or intra-ocular. A retrobulbar injection is usually into the extraocular muscles, or the tissues surrounding these muscles but, in very special cases, retrobulbar injections are deliberately made into the optic nerve. Other very special forms of parenteral injections include epidural, (intra-)medullary and intrathecal.

MONITORING THE ADMINISTRATION of PHARMACEUTICALS

In clinical practice, the administration of pharmaceuticals can be carried out in a variety of ways. These include pill counting, the use of date-marked dispensing devices, and fixed volume or unit dispensing devices with special tamper-proof closures. When a drug is being tested in clinical trials, details of the pharmacokinetics are obtained by urine or blood analysis at various times after administration of the pharmaceutical.

THE REASONS FOR USE OF DIFFERENT ADMINISTRATION ROUTES and PHARMACEUTICALS

The reason for the many different routes of administration of pharmaceuticals is to optimise drug delivery. The different routes of administration are used to take maximum benefit of the natural circulation of drug throughout the body after the pharmaceutical has been administered. Some of the reasons are obvious, e.g. in local therapy of diseases or ailments, it is logical to apply a skin ointment to an abrasion, to spray decongestants up the nose or use eye drops to relieve irritation of the conjunctiva. However, for drug delivery to the inside of the body, the different routes are designed to optimise drug delivery to the target organ. This optimisation is primarily related to the metabolism (biotransformation) of drugs in the human body. This metabolism (break down) of drugs primarily occurs in the liver. Most medications are taken by the oral route and, as a result, are usually readily metabolised by the liver because the circulation around the GI tract leads straight to the liver (via the hepatic portal system). As a result, a certain percentage of the absorbed drug (10 to 99 %) is metabolised by the liver within minutes of being absorbed into the body; this process is called *first-pass metabolism*. When deciding how much drug is needed to manage any disease in the body, this first-pass metabolism has to be taken into account (and that is why the pharmacokinetics are so important). However, first-pass metabolism can be largely avoided if the conjunctival, buccal, sublingual, nasal, rectal and vaginal modes of administration are used because the drug initially enters the peripheral circulation and then moves to the main circulation before then going to the liver. This avoidance of first pass metabolism means that drugs systemically absorbed after conjunctival delivery can have substantial systemic effects.

There are many reasons for the use of different pharmaceuticals. Some of these reasons are simply so that the actual mode of administration can be effected (see above). However, there are also other reasons relating to optimisation of drug delivery for a particular mode of administration. For example, a normal tablet is designed to dissolve slowly in the stomach fluids and any drug administered orally has to be stable both to oral digestive enzymes and to the acid pH of the stomach. The same drug has to also be soluble in either gastric or duodenal fluids in order to be effectively absorbed into the body after oral administration. However, if the tablet is coated, or is a slow- / sustained-release tablet or caplet, then the dissolution will not occur until the pharmaceutical is about to leave the stomach. As a result, the drug release is either slow (and thus non-irritating to the stomach), or timed such that it occurs just as the drug enters the lower alimentary tract. In marked contrast, parenteral administration is generally used to allow administration of a drug that cannot be administered orally (because it is unstable, e.g. insulin) or because it is necessary to get a drug into the tissues or circulation very rapidly.

DRUG BIOTRANSFORMATION (METABOLISM)

After pharmaceuticals are administered, the drugs in these pharmaceuticals are circulated round the body, and are then biotransformed and then excreted. Some form of metabolism (biotransformation) is often necessary before a drug is excreted as its metabolite (especially via the urine). The drug metabolism usually initially results in a break-down of the drug into an inactive metabolite, and thus this process is termed non-synthetic biotransformation. As a second step, most initial drug metabolites are then metabolised further to change them into a chemical form that is optimum for excretion from the body. This second stage is usually termed synthetic biotransformation because the drug is derivatised as a result of chemical side chains being added to the drug, e.g. methylation, acetylation etc.

The non-synthetic biotransformation of a drug by the tissues of the body does not always have to result in its inactivation. Some metabolites (as well as the initial drug) have biological activity. In addition, some pharmaceuticals are specially designed such that the drug has no biological activity until it is biotransformed by the body. These are the *pro-drugs* and they constitute a very important aspect of modern pharmaceuticals. Drugs may be used in the pro-drug form to change the taste of a drug, to increase stability, to increase bioavailability (due to increased tissue penetration) or to allow site-specific delivery to cells or tissues in the body.

DRUG BIOELIMINATION (EXCRETION) FROM THE BODY

(**a**) via the kidney. The kidney excretion route (i.e. renal excretion) is generally the most important route for drug excretion. The substantial part (70 %) of most drugs are eliminated from the body by this route. If a patient has kidney malfunction, drug excretion is thus likely to be impaired and such patients are at risk for development of adverse effects from having too much residual drug in their bodies. Drugs that promote urinary output (diuretics) can increase bioelimination, and *vice versa*.

(**b**) via biliary and fecal routes. Many drug metabolites are secreted into the intestinal tract via the bile fluids (through the spleen). After such internal excretion, these metabolites are eliminated in the feces along with orally administered drugs that were never actually absorbed into the body. If absorbed and metabolised, the drug products are originally produced in the liver hepatocytes / ducts and then transferred to the bile system, rather than simply being transferred via the blood to the kidney, or rest of the body.

Not all orally-administered "medicines" are even intended for absorption. Such non-absorption is known as "non-systemic" drug delivery, e.g. the cholestyramine resins that are given concurrent with other medicines to promote fecal elimination of cholesterol. The resin is eliminated in the feces.

(**c**) via the tears. A little studied phenomenon but can occur, and can be a cause of ocular irritation, e.g. some systemic anti-cancer drugs such as cytarabine are eliminated in the tears and can cause a toxic conjunctivitis.

(**d**) via breast milk. Clinically, one should assume that any drug administered to a nursing mother can be transferred to her milk, and thus to her child; these drugs may be hazardous to the infant. Modern-day pharmaceutical directories (e.g. MIMS or equivalent) ever more frequently contain statements as to whether the drugs in question should be taken by a nursing mother, and such precautions apply to both P and PoM products. The use of many medicines is thus not recommended for nursing mothers, but there are very important exceptions, e.g. anti-epilepsy drugs such as phenytoin need to be taken for the "well-being" of mother and child.

(**e**) in the hair and skin. Pigmented skin is more likely to accumulate drugs and their metabolites. Assessments of hair and skin samples can be used medically or in forensic sciences. A sustained accumulation of drugs in the skin or conjunctiva can precipitate photosensitisation reactions, e.g. tetracycline or nalidixic acid (antibiotics) or phenothiazines such as chlorpromazine (used for psychoses / severe anxiety).

(**f**) via the saliva and sweat. Small quantities of drugs and their metabolites can be excreted via these fluids. The quantities will depend on the magnitude of these physiological phenomena in a particular patient; if a drug promoted salivation or sweating as well, then more drug is likely to be eliminated via these routes.

Entero-hepatic shunting. The route of bioelimination of drugs from the body may change according to overall health, and / or the presence of other drugs. Furthermore, even if a drug or its metabolite is secreted in the bile after biotransformation in the liver, these metabolites can still be re-absorbed back into the body and enter the blood stream again. These metabolites might then be excreted via the kidney or another route. In chronic drug dosing, a unique phenomenon can occur, in some patients, even when normal excretion mechanisms appear to be operative. Some drugs readily undergo first- pass metabolism in the liver to produce active metabolites, e.g. digoxin (used for heart attacks), corticosteroids such as hydrocortisone (used for severe inflammation), and phenothiazines. These metabolites are secreted into the alimentary (gastro-intestinal) tract via the bile along with some of the original drug. The secreted drug and metabolites are then re-absorbed into the body and are re-cycled back to the liver for another round of transformation and secretion; this cycling can go on for days to weeks and is called entero-hepatic shunting. It can result in most unwanted and sustained medicinal effects, or ADR's that can persist for a long time after the medication has been discontinued.

OPHTHALMIC PHARMACEUTICALS

Purpose of chapter. Ophthalmic pharmaceuticals are very special pharmaceuticals designed for topical (ocular) use or application. As specialists in eye diagnosis and care, optometrists need to have a detailed knowledge and understanding of these pharmaceuticals so as to be able to answer any questions on them, as well as to use them appropriately. It is the goal of this chapter to provide this knowledge and understanding, as well as details of the terminologies for ingredients of ophthalmic pharmaceuticals.

Every *pharmaceutical* that is legitimately marketed through regular pharmacists should be dispensed in an approved form and container and have some details of what is in the product - beyond the actual "active" ingredient. The pharmaceutical companies are required to state what the active drug is in a pharmaceutical, and are encouraged to give some details of the other ingredients. A product might be encountered that neither has details of its ingredients, nor are those details to be found in a pharmaceutical directory; try to avoid using such products, as the risks far outweigh the potential benefit. Similarly, the use of any product that does not clearly have a UK license (label) should be approached cautiously.

OPHTHALMIC PHARMACEUTICAL PRODUCTTYPES (PRESENTATION) AND THEIR USE

(1) <u>Solutions</u> marketed in single use containers (e.g. MINIMS^R, or equivalent), also known as SDU's (single dose units). Most containers are made of clear plastic with a snap-off top or cap. Such single-use containers are considered ideal for diagnostic drug use in an optometric practice, and should be selected wherever possible. While referred to as "unit dose", these single-use containers can contain up to 7 drops of solution but are <u>always</u> be for single-use only (and then be discarded immediately).

(2) <u>Solutions</u> or <u>suspensions</u> are usually marketed in 2.5 to 15 mL plastic bottles with screw caps covering a specially designed nozzle/dropper tip (e.g. a DROP-TAINER^R). A few products consist of a bottle with screw cap with the cap being fitted with an "eye dropper" pipette, and some new products are in plastic ampoules with caps. The plastic for the bottles is usually clear, but may be opaque or white if the pharmaceutical is considered to be light sensitive (although not all light-sensitive pharmaceuticals are packaged in opaque containers). Bottle caps may be colour-coded or have a number/day dial incorporated into them (e.g. C-CAP™). Some hospitals may use a special spray dispenser for solutions (e.g. cycloplegics). Products are designed for multiple use <u>by a single individual</u> or for multiple use/users by eye / health care professionals. <u>All</u> such products really should be disposed of after 4 weeks of use, even if the packaging (sometimes) recommends otherwise.

(**3**) <u>Ointments</u> or <u>gels</u> marketed in aluminum (foil) tubes usually containing 3 to 5 gm of material, but can be up to 10 gm. Tubes are closed with a screw cap, that may be colour-coded. The products are designed for multiple use <u>by a single individual</u> or multiple use/users by eye / health care professionals. <u>All</u> multi-use ophthalmic ointments should be discarded after one month.

(**4**) <u>Wafers or inserts</u> marketed in sterile external packaging in which the drug is impregnated into the pharmaceutical form; for single use only.

2. THE PHARMACEUTICAL VEHICLE

The <u>vehicle</u> for a drug is the basis for classification of ophthalmic pharmaceutical types. Even if of the same type (e.g. solutions), most pharmaceuticals are slightly or substantially different from each other. The <u>vehicle</u> is the proper term to describe the delivery system in which the drug is dissolved or dispersed, e.g. aqueous or oil solutions etc.

NOTE. The vehicle does not dictate the mode of administration of the pharmaceutical. It is commonplace to <u>instill</u> eye drops into the lower cul-de-sac, <u>apply</u> ointments onto the conjunctival surface or to the lid margin, and <u>apply</u> or <u>touch</u> a dry wafer to the conjunctival surface. Other modes of administration of these pharmaceuticals are also acceptable. Solutions could be <u>applied</u> ("painted") onto the corneal or conjunctival surface with a sterile cotton bud applicator (e.g. Q-TIP™), a fluorescein strip could be moistened with a drop of a topical anaesthetic or sterile saline prior to insertion into the lower cul-de-sac or application to the conjunctiva, or a solution or ointment could be applied to the lids with a sterile cotton bud applicator.

(**a**) <u>Aqueous solutions</u>. Products formulated for use as eye drops or as irrigating solutions usually can be expected to have an <u>osmolality</u> (tonicity) similar to tears (i.e. are considered as isotonic with tears, ~300 mOsm/L). Hypotonic solutions (240 mOsm/L) are generally well tolerated by the eye, but hypertonic solutions tend to elicit a marked stinging solution on instillation!. Aqueous solutions will usually have a <u>pH</u> value that is considered to be the same or similar to tears (i.e. 7.0 to 7.4). A few products have to be formulated outside of this range (e.g. pH 5.0) simply because they are so unstable at neutral pH. Acidic also solutions tend to elicit a marked stinging solution on instillation.

(**b**) <u>Ophthalmic suspensions</u>. An aqueous vehicle into which is added very small particles of a therapeutic drug. The particles may be generally amorphous (e.g. a flocculated suspension) or be of a very specific size (e.g. microfine nano-particles). To ensure the desired clinical effect is to be achieved, the former products must be well shaken just before use while the latter products should be lightly shaken just before use.

(**c**) <u>Ophthalmic gels</u>. A special polymer (a viscous "solution) that slowly disperses in the tear film (or can be a solution that forms a gel on mixing with the tear film) which forms a film across the ocular surface that is essentially transparent. While having greatly improved optical qualities with respect to ointments, analyses of clinical use suggests that not all eyes will tolerate gels. Some discomfort or smeary vision can result, or a mild "toxic" keratitis can develop with repeated use of the pharmaceutical. The latter may either be due to the gel, the fact that the formulations are rather acidic (*c*. pH 6.0) or the simple fact that drugs in the gel now have prolonged contact with the corneal surface.

(**d**) <u>Ophthalmic ointments</u>. A mixture of a petrolatum base (referred to as white or yellow petrolatum) with wool fat, with or without <u>lanolin</u>. The material is "greasy" and has limited miscibility with the tear film. It has to be stable at room temperature for storage, although some ointments require refrigeration because the drug (or the drug-ointment dispersion) is unstable at room temperature. Most ointments, while extremely effective from a therapeutic perspective, suffer from being "messy" and have the potential for slightly reducing visual acuity.

(**e**) <u>Ophthalmic wafers</u> (or strips). These can either be made of a fibrous material similar to filter paper (and not dissimilar to a Schirmer strip) that is impregnated with a drug, usually a diagnostic drug (e.g. fluorescein or Lissamine green). On being moistened (e.g. with tears on contact with the eye *or* a drop of sterile saline or equivalent) the drug very rapidly washes out. An alternative, marketed in the UK from 1993-1996, was the NODS[R] (new ophthalmic delivery system) in which the drug (tropicamide) was impregnated into a special "plastic" lamellae to be moistened by the tears to effect drug delivery. All such products must be stored dry.

(**f**) <u>Oil (solutions)</u>. A highly purified fraction of vegetable oils (e.g. castor oil, peanut oil) chosen such that it is very fluid at body temperature (the ocular surface is considered to be at 33 to 34°C rather than 37.5°C) and has good light transmission properties even though it may be slightly "coloured" (e.g. slightly yellow).

(**g**) <u>Ophthalmic inserts</u> (4 types).

(i) **Ocusert**[TM] Pilo. This is small insoluble contact lens-like object. It's size is approx. 13.5 mm by 5.5 mm and is 0.3 mm thick. It is placed in the lower cul-de-sac. It has a special membrane that is impregnated with drug such that it will be very slowly washed out of by the tears over a period of 7 days. After this time, the insert is removed from the lower cul-de-sac, discarded, and replaced with another. Product must be stored in a refrigerator. The same principle was used for ophthalmic lamellae many years ago (c. 1900).

(b) Contact lenses (soft) or collagen shields pre-soaked in eye drops. The medicated bandage lens principle. These are soaked in a drug solution (e.g. an antibiotic) for 30 min and then inserted into the eye; the drug is then released over the next 1 to 2 hours (not days).

(c) intra-scleral inserts. These devices are implanted through the conjunctiva into the sclera and should slowly release drugs into the eye, e.g. ganciclovir implants (**Vitrasert**™) for CMV retinitis.

(d) LACRISERT™ (not marketed in UK) is an insert made of 5 mg of hydroxypropylcellulose and contains no other ingredients. It is placed in the lower cul-de-sac. It slowly dissolves in the lacrimal fluid of the lower cul-de-sac over a period of several hours.

3. STABILITY AND STERILITY OF OPHTHALMIC PHARMACEUTICALS.

Ophthalmic pharmaceuticals should only be prepared by pharmaceutical companies or an approved (hospital) pharmacy service. Ophthalmic pharmaceuticals have various types of vehicles which, by law, have to be stable and sterile at the time of being dispensed, sold, opened etc., and meet certain formulation requirements. In order to meet these requirements, ophthalmic pharmaceuticals are prepared under very controlled conditions using extremely pure solvents and chemicals. The requirements for stability and sterility are specified in terms of the labelled content of the active ingredient (drug) and, to a lesser extent, all other ingredients. An ophthalmic pharmaceutical should meet these stability and sterility requirements up to the limit of the expiration date on the actual product. Once the product is opened, the user (practitioner, patient etc.) is responsible for taking reasonable care of the product in such a way that the stability and sterility are maintained. The stability issue primarily addresses the active ingredient, while issues of sterility primarily address the vehicle (although a microbe-contaminated product is more likely to be unstable in terms of the active ingredient, and the presence of an unstable preservative in a product could increase the chance of loss of sterility of the product).

The STABILITY of an ophthalmic pharmaceutical is determined primarily by its pH. This pH is that at which the drug(s) show the slowest rate of chemical breakdown. Most pharmaceuticals have some "pH adjusters" added (e.g. small amounts of acid or alkali added to adjust the pH). In order to achieve a stable pH, the chemicals that are used to give the solution the required pH need to be stable. Simple solutions of NaCl (saline) containing phosphate-, acetate- or borate buffers are very stable, but solutions containing carbonate or bicarbonate are less stable. The stability is also influenced by the osmolality (sometimes referred to as tonicity) of a   . solution. The osmolality can only be maintained if the bottle cap is kept on. The actual concentration of the active ingredient(s) in a pharmaceutical also are important in determining that the specified drug concentration it is within certain limits and remains that way. The active ingredient should thus be stable in its vehicle, and with all of the other ingredients and additives. If commercials products are diluted, they may then be unstable, so such a practice is <u>not</u> recommended (unless done by a hospital pharmacy).

In order to ensure that these stability requirements are realised, a pharmaceutical has a specified <u>shelf life</u> (i.e. the time period between the manufacture and the expiration date). Definition of stability is usually that the pharmaceutical always contains within 10 % of the specified concentration (e.g. 1 % w/v, which is 1 g/100 mL or 10 mg/mL) at the time of manufacture and right up to the expiration date, regardless of whether the product was opened or not. Such requirements can only be realised if the product is appropriately stored and used. Depending in their stability, different ophthalmic products have different a shelf life; a very stable product could be manufactured and be usable for 3 yr. (a long shelf life, e.g. most mydriatics and cycloplegics) while other moderately stable products may only have a shelf life of 1 yr. (e.g. most ophthalmic topical anaesthetics). Most ophthalmic products can be stored at room temperature (8 to 25°C) but some must be kept refrigerated (4°C) to meet this shelf life (e.g. any eye drops containing chloramphenicol). Shelf-life is not the only issue in determining stability of an ophthalmic pharmaceutical since, at some time, the seals on the pharmaceutical will be broken as it opened for use. Thus, especially for some pharmaceuticals, it is necessary to consider a <u>usage life</u> once opened (i.e. once opened, how long are the contents of the bottle or tube stable?). Most ophthalmic products are reasonably stable once opened providing the container is kept closed; this stability may be achieved through the use of "stabilisers" (see below). Some pharmaceuticals may however be rather unstable, they have a short usage life and should be kept refrigerated and used within a very short time period after opening (e.g. ophthalmic solutions containing the antibiotic chloramphenicol should be refrigerated and used within 21 days).

The STERILITY of an ophthalmic pharmaceutical means that it contains zero bacteria or any other microorganisms or their metabolic products etc., including pyrogens, etc., at the time of manufacture. The initial sterility should be maintained up to the expiration date and is achieved by sterile preparation of the pharmaceutical(s) that should only be carried out in special facilities and using special equipment. Ophthalmic pharmaceuticals should also maintain their sterility once opened (providing they are used according to manufacturers recommendations). If the pharmaceutical is intended for multiple use, it should be resistant to significant colonisation by bacteria or other microorganisms. A general guideline exists in the UK in that it is recommended that all multiple use containers of ophthalmic products should be discarded 1 month after opening; the labels of some contact lens re-wetting solutions however (still) state that the products can be used for up to 6 months after opening (not recommended). The recommendation is designed to minimize the chance of products becoming significantly contaminated. In practical terms, this means that the multi-use pharmaceutical should contain enough anti-microbial agent(s) (i.e. preservatives) to ensure an almost instantaneous elimination of any active pathogens for any reasonable level of contamination with bacteria etc. Only preservatives can effectively guarantee this resistance to pathogen growth, although some other ingredients have some bacteriostatic action (e.g. EDTA and some surfactant polymers such as polysorbate 80 or poloxamer). The pathogen elimination from a pharmaceutical is assessed by a "kill curve". The number of viable organisms is assessed as function of time and a time, in minutes, to a 50 % kill (LD_{50}) or the 90 % kill (LD_{90}) determined.

C. STABILISERS and STERILITY-PRESERVING AGENTS.

In order for these goals of stability and sterility to be realised, ophthalmic pharmaceuticals commonly contain -

(**a**) stabilisers. Some active ingredients (drugs) require the continuous presence of another chemical to ensure that they remain in the state in which they were manufactured. Stabilisers reduce the oxygen-dependent degradation of the active ingredient, e.g. topical ocular anaesthetics. Commonly used stabilisers include sodium metabisulphite (often referred to as bisulphites), low concentrations of N-acetylcysteine, or low concentrations of EDTA (also called disodium edetate, edetate sodium or even sodium versenate).

(**b**) preservatives. A common ingredient in ophthalmic pharmaceuticals and necessary for any product marketed in a bottle or a tube intended for multiple use, unless very special precautions were to be taken during use. Several different preservatives are used, but benzalkonium chloride is the commonest. This quaternary ammonium compound is a cationic compound with surface-active (surfactant) properties and is usually included at concentrations of 0.01 % or less. Cetrimide (also known as cetrimonium or cetyltrimethylammonium bromide), polidronium chloride (POLYQUAD^R) and benzododecinium bromide are also quaternary ammonium cationic surfactants being more widely used nowadays, and probably at concentrations of 0.001 to 0.01 %. Another cationic surfactant is benzethonium chloride, but is rarely used. All these "quaternary ammonium" surfactants disrupt the cell membranes of microorganisms and can be bacteriostatic or bactericidal depending on the concentration used. Another common alternative preservative is chlorbutol [also known as chlor(o)butanol], a chloroform-like alcohol that perturbs cell membranes, and included at the 0.5 % concentration. A similar compound to chlorbutol is phenylethyl alcohol, while myrisyl-gamma-picolinlum chloride is an alkyl-substituted benzyl alcohol. Chlorhexidine is a non-ionic biguanide alkyl ammonium compound that also perturbs cell membranes at the 0.005 to 0.01 % concentration. An older group of chemicals are simply non-specifically toxic to microorganisms. These include the organomercurials such as thiomersal (also known as thimerosal) probably included at concentrations of 0.01 to 0.02 %, while others such as phenylmercuric nitrate or acetate are now rarely used. A range of benzoic acid derivatives such as p-hydroxybenzoate, parabens, methyl-parabens or propyl-parabens can be found in ointments (but the concentrations are rarely specified). NOTE that in contact lens saline solutions, soaking, disinfectant or cleaning solutions, some other bacteriostatic or bactericidal chemicals can be found. These include sorbic acid, DYMED^R (another quaternary ammonium compound, that is sometimes referred to by its chemical name of polyaminopropyl biguanide), chlorhexidine, polyhexanide and related compounds, alkyl triethanol ammonium chloride (another quaternary ammonium compound), phenoxyethanol, benzyl alcohol, and a range of chloride-generating compounds [e.g. halazone (Aerotab^R), and Purite^R].

NOTE on contact lens use and ophthalmic pharmaceuticals. Other than the bandage lens principle (see above), the only eyedrops that should really be used while a contact lens is in place are contact lens re-wetting solutions (see Chapter 11). Current recommendations are generally that any other preservative-containing eyedrop should not be used "whilst or imediately before wearing (soft) contact lenses". Five minutes should be a sufficient interval between instilling eyedrops and re-inserting contact lenses. For a while, the listings of many pharmaceuticals in the directories (e.g. MIMS) included (C/I) contact lenses, or contact lens wear or soft contact lenses. This can be generally viewed as a precautionary measure to limit the chance of a toxic keratitis developing when, for example, benzalkonium chloride-containing eyedrops were used concurrently with soft lens wear.

4. POLYMERS / VISCOLISERS

Ophthalmic pharmaceuticals work best when they are stable and sterile. However, providing this stability and sterility means that many eye drops also produce a slight irritation when instilled, and reflex lacrimation occurs. Polymers are therefore widely used in eye drops to slow down the rapid wash out caused by reflex lacrimation (and thus improve drug delivery to the eye). These polymers should be unreactive with all ingredients of the eyedrops. Most polymers are classified as "viscolisers", i.e. these polymers increase the viscosity of the eye drops, making them less watery, e.g. cellulose polymers (e.g. hypromellose, hydroxyethylcellulose etc), polyvinyl alcohol (= PVA), glycerol (also known as glycerine), polyvinylpyrollidone (also known as povidone or polyvidone), polyethylene glycol (abbreviated as PEG), dextran 40 or 80, carbowax, poloxamer 407, polysorbate or carbomers (e.g Carbomer 934 or 940, also known as polyacrylic acid). A newer viscoliser is gellan gum (that makes a very viscous solution).

5. EXCIPIENTS (other ingredients)

Eyedrops can, by law, contain a number of other "inactive" ingredients. These include various natural oils and plant extracts.

6. LIMITS OF USE OF OPHTHALMIC PHARMACEUTICALS

The LABEL on all pharmaceuticals should be checked immediately before use !. All ophthalmic products should carry the proprietary (brand) name either on an affixed label or stamped into the plastic wrap of a single-use container. On single-use products, the name may be abbreviated, e.g. TRO 1.0 stands for tropicamide 1.0 % on a Minims[R] product.

All ophthalmic pharmaceuticals will have an expiration date. For the multi-use pharmaceuticals, this is most commonly stamped onto the labelling of the bottle or tube. For unit-dose / single use pharmaceuticals, this is most commonly an impression stamped into the plastic or foil of the container. Vials carry a label or, occasionally, a date etched into the glass. The expiration date is the last day of the month indicated (e.g. EXP SEP 99). No pharmaceutical should ever be used AFTER the expiration date, even one day after. It is important that expiration dates be taken into account during storage and stocktaking. Some type of stock rotation is essential to ensure that older stocks get used first and newer stocks get used after the ones with an earlier expiration date. Just because stocks were received more recently does not mean however that they have a later expiration date and it is the stock-takers responsibility to check!. If pharmaceuticals have never been opened and reach their expiry date, they should still be discarded.

Ophthalmic pharmaceuticals will have a batch (= lot) number as they are prepared in batches (e.g. thousands of individual bottles / tubes from a single stock of a solution or ointment, etc.). Each of these batches will have a unique number assigned to it (e.g. LOT2J). The batch number is usually found on the label of the product alongside the expiration date. It is not usually necessary to record the batch number when using pharmaceuticals although, in a large practice, stock-taking / inventory might include details of these. However, the batch number is important whenever an adverse reaction occurs or is thought to be associated with the use of any ophthalmic pharmaceutical; the marketing or distributing company will want to know from which lot the suspect pharmaceutical came from.

ALL pharmaceuticals should be inspected immediately before use. Degraded solutions may show a slight or substantial colour change (e.g. yellow or even orange brown in rare cases for ophthalmic anaesthetic solutions), or contain fine to coarse precipitates. Since almost all ophthalmic solutions (as opposed to suspensions) are clear and colorless solutions, the presence of any significant colour or precipitates can be easily assessed with the "white tile" test (i.e. applying several drops of a solution onto white tissue that has been folded over several times). Exceptions include some ophthalmic solutions which are already   slightly coloured (e.g. nedocromil sodium or pilocarpine solutions), or ophthalmic suspensions (that can look slightly cloudy). Notwithstanding, it is also important to consider the possibility of contamination of ophthalmic pharmaceuticals, especially for products brought in by patients. Microbe-contaminated pharmaceuticals are very difficult to identify. The contaminated solution may well have a high enough pathogen count to be able to deliver a significant dose of viable pathogens to the ocular surface but still be almost clear and colourless. It is unlikely there would be much change in the appearance or consistency of an ophthalmic ointment even when there was a substantial bacterial count. Therefore, one has to largely rely on external signs on the container. Any indication that a solution does not "look right" is cause enough for it to be discarded. If there are any deposits or encrustation around the bottle tip or tube nozzle, the chance of contamination is high. Such products should be discarded, even if, for example, a patient still wishes to keep them for use.

Access to all pharmaceuticals should be restricted. It is a very bad practice to leave pharmaceuticals lying around. Any type of ophthalmic pharmaceutical should not be left lying around on counter tops etc. either in an optometric office or at home. These products can end up in the hands of children, or in the hands of the patients who definitely should not have them (e.g. topical anesthetics taken by patients with irritated or painful eyes).

Pharmaceuticals should always be kept closed and should NEVER be left with their cap or closure off; this includes contact lens saline solutions !. Bottle caps, etc. should always be returned to their container immediately after drops have been dispensed etc., and closures replaced on containers of tablets, etc. This applies to in-office and well as home (domiciliary) use.

Contamination of the delivery system of the ophthalmic pharmaceuticals should be avoided. Every reasonable effort should routinely be made to prevent such contamination of the ophthalmic eye drop bottle tip or cap (or ointment tube nozzle, etc.) either with fingers or non-sterile tissue. Bottle caps that have fallen on the floor etc., should not be placed back on bottles, tubes etc. When instilling eye drops, any contact with the patients eyelashes, lid skin, conjunctiva etc. should be avoided. The application of ophthalmic ointments may preferably be done with a sterile cotton bud applicator rather than touching the nozzle to the eyelid margins or ocular surface. Some recommend that a half-inch ribbon be ejected and discarded from ophthalmic ointment tubes prior to each use on the eye.

7. STORAGE OF PHARMACEUTICALS

(a) temperature. Pharmaceuticals should be stored as far as possible according to the manufacturers instructions. Most ophthalmic pharmaceuticals can be stored at room temperature (8 to 25°C) but it is important to check the small print on the label. The recommended conditions of storage are specific for the pharmaceutical and not always for the active ingredients *per se*. In most cases, several simple rules can be adopted. Avoid storing any pharmaceutical at temperatures above an expected upper limit of 30°C, but most pharmaceuticals do not need to be stored in a refrigerator. There are a few exceptions that should be stored at 4°C and include some topical ocular anaesthetics or phenylephrine solutions, eyedrops containing chloramphenicol, reconstituted solutions of echothiophate, viscous eye drops of latanoprost, and the **Ocusert**[R] ophthalmic inserts (containing pilocarpine). A note that states 'refrigerate at 4°C' should be taken literally - it does not mean the ice box / freezer compartment of the refrigerator !. For shorter periods of time, including their use during the working day, at least ensure that these pharmaceuticals that should be refrigerated (e.g. topical ocular anaesthetics) are kept cool (10 to 20°C). A designated (4°C) pharmaceuticals refrigerator should be available for large quantities of perishable pharmaceutical products. It is never good practice to store "drugs" with the beverages, lunch, etc.

(b) lighting. Even brief periods of exposure to very high intensity lighting, or prolonged exposure to even standard office lighting, should be avoided if the product has a clear plastic container; opaque plastic bottles offer some light protection and amber glass bottles do the same. Glass front display cases are acceptable only if the pharmaceuticals are kept in the cardboard cartons they were dispensed in OR when the use of the pharmaceutical is so substantial that a bottle or unit dose product would only be on the shelf or a week or so.

(c) humdity. High humidity should be avoided. This is only really essential for ophthalmic wafers (fluorescein or rose bengal strips). However, high humidity means that there is an increased chance for adherence of dust etc.. For the patient at home or travelling, the following are useful tips, especially for those on chronic medication. Locations such as bathroom "medicine" cabinets are great for many o.t.c. care products (soap, shampoo, toothpaste etc.), but are rarely good places to keep ophthalmic pharmaceuticals. Car glove boxes or the boot are never good places to leave ophthalmic pharmaceuticals and airplane luggage holds may not be suitable for some pharmaceuticals (because of temperature extremes and lack of accessibility) and it is best that they are carried in hand luggage.

Other issues that are important relate to access. "Convenient" places for storage of pharmaceuticals should be avoided and this includes the pockets of an optometrist's white coat !. Ophthalmic pharmaceuticals are not generally designed to be carried around. Office clothing or general clothing (pockets etc.) are never good places to keep ophthalmic pharmaceuticals; multiple-use containers can accumulate dust and pathogens far more easily, while these and unit dose/ single use products can also be exposed to uncertain extremes of temperature, humidity etc.

EYEWASHES, OPHTHALMIC DYES, STAINS
and TOPICAL OCULAR ANAESTHETICS

Purpose of chapter. Drug delivery to the eye is a complex process. The time base of action of drugs on the eye is determined by this delivery process, and the mechanisms underlying it. The purpose of this chapter is to explain these mechanisms and to illustrate them by considering the actions of eyewashes, dyes and stains and topical ocular anesthetics.

After presentation of solutions, eyedrops, gels or ointments to the surface of the eye, a series of time-dependent changes can be expected to occur. Ocular *pharmacokinetics* is a quantitative description of the time base of drug action on the eye, i.e. is a description of the delivery and wash-out of a drug from the eye. Pharmacokinetics allows one to compare the effects of any drugs on the eye, and includes those effects following the use of eyewashes, diagnostic or therapeutic drugs. The pharmacokinetics has two components - a description of the time base (i.e. how fast or how slow, and how long an effect is) and the magnitude (i.e. how big or how small the effect is and is it an increase or a decrease).

TOPICAL OCULAR PHARMACEUTICALS and their effects

After an eye drop is instilled into the lower cul-de-sac, several inter-related steps occur in a normal eye. Firstly, the solution mixes with the tear film. However, almost immediately after the mixing, rapid drainage from the cul-de-sac will start to occur (unless special measures are taken; see later) so that most of the solution will be washed down the naso-lacrimal duct and is ultimately be absorbed into the body via the nasal mucosa and vasculature. Only a small proportion (< 5 %) of the solution (and any drugs dissolved in it) is thus available for absorption by the ocular tissues. This absorption occurs both into the corneal epithelium and the conjunctival epithelium. Only very small quantities (< 1 % of initial dose) actually enter the eye. After absorption, the ingredients of the solution can diffuse through into the anterior chamber of the eye. Some of the eye drop is absorbed into the conjunctival tissue and conjunctival vasculature to either enter the peripheral circulation or actually diffuse into the anterior or posterior chamber of the eye. Any ingredients of the eye drop that actually entered the eye will then later be eliminated from the intra-ocular compartment (following aqueous humour flow) to then enter the systemic circulation. It should be noted that even after absorption, not all of the drug is available to effect clinical responses.

Melanin pigment may bind some drugs quite extensively so that some of the drug (having entered the eye) is non-specifically adsorbed onto the pigment and is thus not available to bind to receptors (e.g. those on iris muscles); a later slow release can then produce prolonged effects.

For many ophthalmic products, it will take just a few minutes for some drug absorption into the cornea to occur, and about 30 to 60 min before the maximum concentration in the aqueous humour is achieved. In the normal lens-containing (phakic) eye, there is usually no measurable diffusion of the drug past the crystalline lens and into the vitreous. However, after cataract operations, some of the drugs in eye drops can diffuse through the vitreous to the retina (but without clinical consequences in most cases).

A modern-day eye drop usually has a volume of about 35 ul. This volume is larger than that which can be retained on the ocular surface so an initial fast wash-out of the solution occurs. If this is down the naso-lacrimal duct, it will depend on the patency of the puncta and naso-lacrimal ducts, otherwise it will overflow onto the cheeks. The reflex tearing that usually occurs following eye drop instillation (because the eye drops elicit a "stinging" sensation), makes the rates of drug wash-out even faster because the tear volume is even further increased. Crying (e.g. in children) often results in such fast drug wash-out that no drug effects on the eye occur. Instillation of eye drops in quick succession can elicit such reflex tearing that there is little clinical effect, even though several drops were used. However, the rate of this wash-out can be dramatically slowed down by voluntary eye closure or by punctal occlusion. As a result, the quantity of drug that is available for absorption into the eye can be expected to increase. For this reason, after eye drops are used, lid closure is highly recommended rather than letting a patient blink and promote the wash-out process. Just 30s to 60s voluntary eye closure (after eye drop instillation) should significantly enhance drug delivery to the eye. If more than one eye drop is to be used, at least three minutes (and preferably 5 min) should elapse between each drop.

The extent of drug absorption will also be determined by the health of the corneal and conjunctival epithelia. A healthy layer of cells acts as a natural barrier to drug absorption while a compromised tissue will readily absorb drugs (e.g. fluorescein will be absorbed into the cornea far more easily if there is compromise of the corneal surface). Patient age is also an important factor in determining the efficacy of ophthalmic drugs. Age may alter reflex lacrimation, the integrity of the corneal surface may be different in older patients and the tissues in the eye can respond differently to the same drug.

Overall therefore, in order to be able to describe the effects of an eye drop (ointment or gel) on the eye, the drug concentration in the pharmaceutical, the quantity used (e.g. the number of drops instilled, the quantity of ointment applied etc), patient eye colour, and their age need to be specified as well as noting whether the eyelids were closed or left open after instillation etc. With these principles of ocular pharmacokinetics in mind, the clinical reality of these mechanisms can be addressed. These principles can be illustrated by consideration of the effects of eyewashes, dyes, stains and anaesthetics on the eye.

1. EYEWASHES

The use of an ophthalmic wash solution (i.e. an eyewash) should wash debris and the tear film from the ocular surface and then exit via the nasolacrimal duct or overflow onto the peri-ocular skin; eyelid closure is not wanted here because the idea here is to promote wash-out. Eyewash ingredients will usually not have a chance to be absorbed into the ocular tissues. Eyewashes can be used extensively in whatever volume is considered necessary or appropriate. For example, an eyewash may be needed to wash away an ophthalmic dye or stain, gonioscopic gels or to remove allergens. Some of these products do however contain preservatives and thus, with excessive use, could precipitate some irritation / discomfort / mild staining of the cornea due to the preservative; such events are very rare. A special effort should be made to avoid contamination of eyewash solutions, especially if they are being used to relive allergic symptoms or the residuals of a eye infection. When used with an eyecup (see below), this eyecup is only for use by a single individual.

 The simplest eyewash (pharmaceutical) is a sterile saline solution that contains 0.9 % w/v NaCl (sodium chloride, saline) which can be buffered with phosphates or borate / boric acid. A bottle of 150 to 200 mL is the normal quantity supplied but bottles of up to 1000 mL are available. Such solutions (e.g. GSL **Sterac**[R] **Sodium Chloride**) are sterile and available as General Sales List (GSL) Medicines. Small (20 mL) ampules (e.g. GSL **Steri-Wash**[R], GSL **Steripod Blue**[R], or GSL **Sodium Chloride**, generic) or small (25 or 100 mL) foil sachets of sterile saline (e.g. P **Normasol**[R]) are also available. If all that was needed was a small quantity of a saline solution to cleanse the ocular surface (i.e. a mini-eyewash), then sterile saline eye drops in unit-dose eye drops are available (e.g. P **Minims**[R] **Sodium Chloride**), available as Pharmacy Medicines (P).

A contact lens-related sterile saline solution can also be used as an eyewash. These are solutions of 0.9% NaCl or 0.85 % NaCl with a small quantity of added phosphate buffer and are usually preservative-free nowadays because they are dispensed in aerosol canisters (of 100 to 500 mL). These types of solutions are meant to replace a prior practice using salt tablets (or sachets of NaCl powder) and distilled water to prepare eyewashes or solutions for rinsing contact lenses. Commercial products designated as eyewashes are also available off the shelf (as GSL products). These eyewashes, eye salves, eye lotions or eye baths can be sold with an eyecup and usually contain saline with a small quantity of phosphate buffer or are a mixture of boric acid / sodium borate, (e.g. "borate eye wash" or a "solution of borate" used as an eyewash). Bottles of 110 to 200 mL are common sizes. Such solutions usually also contain a small quantity of a preservative such as benzalkonium chloride or thimerosal and also include other ingredients (astringents) designed to promote "cleansing" of the ocular surface. These other ingredients can include chemicals such as witch hazel and glycerin (e.g. as in GSL **Optrex**[R] **Eye Wash / Optrex**[R] **Eye Lotion**, and **Optrex**[R] **Fresh Eyes Wash**™) or flower and plant extracts (e.g. SL **Vital Eyes**™ **Eye Wash**); witch hazel is also known as *Hamamelis* water. Eye drops containing witch hazel (e.g. P **Optrex**[R] **Eye Drop**s, 10 mL or 18 mL; **Fresh Eyes**™ , 10 mL) are available. Single use 15 mL or 10 mL plastic ampoules containing flower and plant extracts (e.g. **Vital Eyes**™) are also available as off-the-shelf, non-medicinal, products. Ampoules of witch hazel (e.g. **I-Doc**[R]) were marketed until recently. An alternative ocular astringent is zinc sulphate 0.25 % (e.g. P **Zinc Sulphate** Eye Drops, generic, 10 mL bottle). More elaborate expensive solutions are used by surgeons to irrigate the eye during operations. A Balanced Salt Solution contains a mixture of salts such as $NaCl$, KCl, $MgCl_2$, $CaCl_2$ and is buffered with acetate and citrate salts. These products are sterile, are marketed in small 15, 18 or 30 mL bottles and are available to professionals as hospital products (e.g. HP **Iocare**[R] **Balanced Salt Solution**, HP **BSS**[R]).

NOTE that in emergencies (e.g. following splashing a chemical in the eye), very large volumes of an eyewash (e.g. GSL **Optrex**[R] **Emergency Eye Wash**, 500 mL) or tap water should be continuously applied for at least 15 min, and preferably longer. A hospital pharmacy may provide **BSS**[R] or equivalent to the emergency room, or their own formulated "buffered eye lotion" (prepared according to recommended British Pharmacopoeia).

2. LID SCRUB PRODUCTS

Lid scrubs is a term used to describe products that are designed to facilitate cleansing of the eyelid margins. Eyelid margin discomfort and decreased tear film instability can develop in cases of (mild-to-moderate) blepharitis or blepharoconjunctivitis, which may be associated with Meibomian gland dysfunction. General surface hygiene measures should reduce the build up of bacteria on the eyelashes, and reduce the chance of other intra-epithelial / glandular / hair follicle infections of the eyelid margin that can develop.

One method of eyelid cleansing is to carefully rub a diluted solution (at least 1:51 v/v) of "baby shampoo" along the eyelid margins once-a-day with a sterile or clean cotton bud applicator. Commercial lid scrub products (e.g. an 80 mL bottle of **LidCare**[R] solution with gauze wipes, or individually-packaged sterile wipes) are designed to replace baby shampoo or other household products (e.g. 3 % w/v bicarbonate of soda) as lid scrubs.

3. SPECIAL IRRIGATION SOLUTIONS.

In some cases, ocular discomfort can be accompanied by oedema (of the cornea or conjunctiva or both) or the irrigation needs to be very aggressive because a toxic chemical has been splashed into the eye. For these situations, some other solutions can also be used.

(a) hypertonic sodium chloride solutions (NaCl, saline, hypertonic) or ointments. May be used as a diagnostic aid, as an astringent, as therapy for corneal epithelial oedema, or as a pre-operative measure. Such solutions are usually used at the 2 % or 5 % concentration of NaCl. There are no commercial products in the UK, but they can be specially prepared by a hospital pharmacy. Their uses are as a <u>diagnostic aid</u> to clear an oedematous corneal epithelium. Several drops may be needed over a period of 15 to 20 min to achieve the desired clearing effect. If the cornea clears, the test was positive for local epithelial oedema (since the water content of the epithelium has been reduced by the hypertonic solution); one can also now see into the eye better with biomicroscopy etc. Hypertonic saline can also be used as an <u>astringent</u> to remove very stringy mucus from dry eyes or following chemical burns (e.g. when symblepharon is present). Hypertonic salines may be used as therapy / <u>periodic relief of corneal oedema</u> (e.g. in a slowly decompensating cornea in cases of bullous keratopathy, including late-stage Fuch's dystrophy patients), an ointment containing high concentrations of NaCl can be used as well here. The hypertonic saline or ointment may serve as <u>therapy for an unstable epithelium</u> after an abrasions or recurrent erosion. Temporary reversal of superficial corneal oedema (associated with such cases) may promote stability to the surface cell layers.

A major hospital may also elect to use other "hypertonics". These can include specially-prepared sterile solutions of glycerin (10 to 50 % v/v diluted with sterile water for irrigation), or even solutions of sucrose or glucose (30 to 40 % w/v). Commercial products containing 40 % glucose (ointments) are available in Europe and the USA.

(b) trisodium edetate (edetate sodium, EDTA, sodium versenate) solutions. These are specially prepared solutions, containing edetate sodium at the 0.37 to 4 % concentration. The EDTA, at high concentrations, inhibits collagenase enzyme activity in the corneal stroma. The EDTA solution can be prepared from a 20 % concentrated solution (generally used for *i.v.* administration; PoM **Limclair**[R]) that is diluted 1: 50 with sterile purified water (by a hospital pharmacy); this is an approved use for "calcareous corneal opacities". These solutions are usually slightly hypertonic and used as an astringent or irrigant for ocular emergencies, especially after alkali (lime) burns to the eye. A common use is after such an eye has been copiously irrigated with tap water in the hospital emergency department. Sodium citrate 10.11 % could be prepared for the same purpose. The EDTA or citrate act as a chelating agent for any divalent cations and so can help remove calcium carbonate or calcium phosphate deposits (that can develop after toxic alkaline solutions have been in the eye) from the ocular surface tissues; will also work as therapy for band keratopathies that develop after systemic calcium imbalance. In such cases, such solutions would be used (by a professional) as an eye salve or eye drops and the application repeated every few days.

NOTE that these uses of concentrated edetate solutions should not be confused with the commonplace use of small quantities (i.e. < 0.1 % w/v, commonly < 0.05 %) of edetate sodium in many eye drops. Here, the edetate sodium has a chelating action that gives the solutions a mild bacteriostatic property (so helps preserve sterility) and confers stability on the solutions (especially for light-sensitive drugs where trace quantities of metals can catalyze photo-degradation).

4. GONIOSCOPIC SOLUTIONS

In applying a gonioscopic lens to the corneal surface, it is generlaly advisable to use some sort of 'cushioning' medium, and this also serves to provide a uniform optical interface between the lens and the eye. While saline can be used, it is preferable to use a more viscous solution, e.g. containing polymers such as hypromellose 1 % (**Isopto**[R] **Alkaline**), or carmellose 1 % unit dose (**Celluvisc**[R]). A hospital pharmacy may prepare small bottles (with a dropper) of hypromellose 1.5 % or equivalent.

5. OPHTHALMIC DYES and STAINS and THEIR USES.

The two terms (dyes and stains) are often used interchangeably; the true origin of the terms for ophthalmic use is obscure and the conditions of use of these agents can determine whether they are simply briefly adding colour to ocular tissue or ocular fluids (=dyes) or whether they are imparting a certain color tinge to the tissue for a number of hours (=stains). The ideal dyes and stains should be fully miscible with the tear film (i.e. be water soluble), and the overall effects should be reversible (especially after use of an eyewash or other irrigant). In reality, the use of fluorescein will leave a patient with orange-yellow coloured lid margins, the use of rose bengal will leave a patient with crimson-coloured lid margins, puncta and conjunctiva.

(**a**) fluorescein sodium solution. Often simply called "fluorescein". It is used in two forms - from paper strips impregnated with the dye (P **Fluorets**[R]) or as eye drops containing the dye (various unit-dose preparations - see below). When dispensed as eye drops, it is an orange-yellow and slightly alkaline, aqueous solution of the sodium salt of fluorescein. The solution also usually also contains a small quantity of buffer (such as borate / boric acid) to stabilise the solution. If the solution also contains an anaesthetic (see below), the pH will be slightly acidic. The fluorescence, as seen under cobalt-blue illumination, is less at slightly acidic pH (i.e. pH 6.8 compared to that at pH 7.4) and the fluorescence may be even greater at pH 7.8. The fluorescence is also concentration- as well as pH-dependent, so that more concentrated films/ pools of the dye will have a greater yellow- green fluorescence than lower concentrations. In all cases however, the fluorescence is intense and is best visualised by using a Wratten #45A filter over the illumination source on the slit lamp, and a Wratten #15 filter over the observation system of the slit lamp. Under these illumination conditions, the fluorescein aids <u>assessments of corneal surface integrity</u> since the dye will tend to pool in areas of the epithelial surface where there are defects and so these show up as highly fluorescent areas. Similarly, when used as an aid for determining the fit of rigid contact lenses, the fluorescein will pool in areas where there is poor fit and be squeezed away from areas where there is contact between the contact lens and the ocular surface. For soft (hydrophilic) contact lenses, a special high MW derivative of fluorescein (fluorexon) is available (P **Fluoresoft**™). Fluorescein is also used as an aid for performing applanation tonometry (usually with anaesthetic) since the applanated area (the "touch" area) will be darker (and purplish-black) compared to the surround. The fact that the fluorescence is proportional to concentration can also be used to assess whether there is a uniform tear film over the ocular surface and to assess whether this tear film is stable. When low concentrations of fluorescein are applied to the eye (i.e. with the fluorescein strip), the tear film will be faintly fluorescent immediately after a full blink; if the film breaks up then dark spots, patches or discontinuities will appear. The time for these to appear is a measure of the stability of the tear film and the procedure is called a tear break up time (TBUT) assessment. Values of less than 10 s are indications of a dry eye. If the patient blinks, the tear film will reform and break up again. If the eye is watched for a minute or so, then the fluorescence in the tear film will be seen to get less and less (especially with each blink); the rate at which this fluorescence declines is a measure of the rate of tear flow since the fluorescein is progressively diluted by the tears. In this case therefore, the fluorescein can be used to assess tear flow. The fluorescein will however only disappear if the lacrimal drainage/ patency is normal. To assess this more reliably, it is best to use larger doses of fluorescein (e.g. 1 or 2 % solution), allow the patient to blink a couple of times, and then perhaps instill a couple of drops of sterile saline before asking a patient to blink again. If the patient then blows their nose into a white tissue, the yellow fluorescein will colour the white tissue if the naso-lacrimal duct is patent. The procedure can be done for the each eye in turn.

The commercially available products that are usually used are the fluorescein-impregnated strips (e.g. P **Fluorets**R that contain 1 mg of the dye) or the sterile unit-dose (single-application) solutions (e.g. P **Minims**R **Fluorescein Sodium** 1 % or 2 %, FLN 1.0 or FLN 2.0). The strips are individually packaged in a sterile paper sleeve and must be stored in a cool, dry place. The MinimsR should be kept in their plastic outer-wrap until used. The special fluorescein polymer, fluorexon (P **Fluoresoft**™), is only about 1/10th as fluorescent as fluorescein sodium; unit dose plastic vials are marketed. Single-use ampoules (sealed glass vials) of sterile fluorescein sodium 10 % or 25 % are used by ophthalmologists in fluorescein angiography of the fundus. These solutions are generally administered i.v. and are not for optometric use.

(**b**) rose bengal ophthalmic solution or strips. Rose bengal is a fluorescein derivative that is used as a "vital" stain in the sense that this crimson-colored chemical appears to be able to bind somewhat selectively and tightly to what are often loosely referred to as devitalized cells of the conjunctival and corneal tissue. It is primarily used as an aid to diagnose a dry eye (see below). Rose bengal also readily stains surface mucus, the lids and puncta (naso-lacrimal ducts). No special illumination system is needed to visualize rose bengal since it is largely non-fluorescent and has a very intense crimson colour that is easily visualized against the white of the eye or even on the corneal surface (when viewed with the slit lamp). After instillation of a drop of the dye (or application of a strip), a patient should be allowed to close their eyes for a few minutes to ensure good staining; the lid closure will tend to lessen any discomfort. A rose bengal-impregnated strip may not easily wet for a patient with substantial lacrimal insufficiency so that inadequate dye may be placed on the ocular surface for a good differential staining. The solution to the problem is to place a drop of sterile saline on the brownish-red tip of the rose bengal strip and then touch this wetted strip to the conjunctiva. The dye, especially as the 1 % solution, can sting quite substantially, although the degree of discomfort could be a useful indicator of the severity of the ocular surface disease. As a result of this irritation, and especially a patient is allowed to keep their eyes open after instillation of rose bengal, then reflex lacrimation will tend to rapidly wash the stain away from the ocular surface. After the staining has been allowed for 3 to 5 minutes, irrigation the eye (with sterile saline or equivalent) is however recommended. This irrigation will remove excess stain, improve resolution and minimize residual staining (especially of the eye lid margins). The irrigation should be done carefully since rose bengal will very readily stain the peri-ocular skin and a patient's clothes !. The use of rose bengal ophthalmic solution is primarily as an aid to detection of chronic ocular surface disease. Examples include keratoconjunctivitis sicca (KCS), exposure keratitis (perhaps associated with keratitis neuroparalytica, non-specific lagophthalmos or exophthalmos). Rose bengal can also be used as a differential diagnosis for true dendritic keratitis (due to herpes virus, where the dendrite-pattern ulcer will stain well with rose bengal) and a pseudodendritic keratitis (due to herpes zoster, where the mucous strands or plaques on the surface will only stain poorly with rose bengal and will not have a pronounced margin as in ulcer lesions).

Rose bengal is usually available in unit dose from as P **Minims**[R] **Rose Bengal** 1 %, and perhaps in small (5 mL) bottles as **Rose Bengal Eye-drops** 1 % (generic). The Minims[R] should be kept in their plastic outer-wraps and preferably stored in a drawer. For the bottles of solution, the stock-and shelf- life is short, and such products may be discontinued at short notice. Rose Bengal strips may also be available (by special import) in a large hospital eye clinic (e.g. **Rosets**[R] or **Rose Bengal Strips**) and should be stored in a cool, dark place at low humidity.

(c) brilliant blue. This is a cobalt blue dye that can be included in eye drops (e.g. P EyeDew[R] Blue) used for cosmesis; a subtle bluish colouration of the conjunctiva can help mask hyperaemia. Methylene blue can be used for the same purpose.

(d) methylene blue ophthalmic solution. This is a bluish-purple dye that can be used as a vital stain, specifically to visualize corneal nerves and any other irregularities of the cornea limbus and conjunctiva. Its commonest use is during surgery where a 1 % solution of the stain is used to mark the sclera or limbus for incision points. However, it can also be used as a general stain for surface lesions if two or three drops of a 0.5 to 1 % solution are used. In ether case, a stain of the conjunctiva (a bluish color) can persist for at least a day. The chemical can also been expected to have mild anti- vasodilatation properties, although this has not been proven for its ophthalmic application.

(e) indocyanine green. This dye is an alternative to fluorescein solutions that are used for angiography, especially of the choroidal circulation or that of the iris. This dye is very unstable in solution so is marketed as a sterile powder that is reconstituted with a special sterile solution immediately before use. It is injected *i.v.*

(e) Lissamine green SF. This non-fluorescein-like dye/ stain (properly known as Green S or Light Green SF) was advocated for conjunctival staining in the 1960's. No commercial products are available in the UK, but it is currently being further evaluated (and products such as Lissamine green strips are avilable in the USA).

6. TOPICAL OCULAR ANAESTHETICS.

Topical ocular anaesthetics are ONLY for use by a professional health care provider on a patient in their office; these anaesthetic solutions are NEVER for self-administration, even by health care providers !. Such use constitutes "abuse" and can lead to very severe, sight-threatening corneal damage.

Topical ocular anaesthetics block nerve conduction and thus stop pain signals being sent from the traumatized or stimulated areas of the ocular surface to the brain. Trauma could be from a foreign body (or its removal) while stimuli include a tonometer probe, a hard or rigid contact lens or gonio-lens, or a naso-lacrimal duct / punctal probe. Topical ocular anaesthetics are thus used as an aid to applanation tonometry (to minimize the sensation of the tonometer probe touching the cornea), as an aid in assessing lacrimal flow (since the anaesthetic will eliminate reflex tearing and leave only basal tear flow), to facilitate examination of an irritated or inflamed eye (since the anesthetic will reduce the sensation of prodding or lid eversion etc.), as an aid in fitting of hard or rigid contact lenses (since the lens fitting may be uncomfortable when performed for the first time) and to permit foreign body removal from the cornea or conjunctiva.

Topical ocular anaesthetics are sometimes referred to as local anaesthetics but this is not a good term. While the same drugs are used for topical ocular anaesthesia and local anaesthesia, the topical ocular anaesthetics are intended solely for anaesthesia of the ocular surface and lid margins as achieved via the instillation of eyedrops; local anaesthetics are generally injected.

For use, a single drop of anaesthetic solution (with or without fluorescein) should be instilled and the patient asked to close their eyes for 15 to 30 s. Alternatively, a fluorescein strip can be wetted with a drop of anaesthetic solution and the wetted strip touched to the conjunctival surface. Excess solution (perhaps squeezed out between the lid margins) can then be wiped away. Topical ocular anaesthetics tend to sting slightly on instillation and promote an initial reflex lacrimation; closing the lids will reduce this stinging effect and reduce anesthetic wash-out. Some anaesthetic eye drops [e.g. proxymetacaine (proparacaine)] are considered more comfortable than others [e.g. amethocaine (tetracaine)].

There are four types of anaesthetics based on their chemical structure -a classification which is important since allergic reactions to anaesthetic drugs are quite common; if they occur, the use of an anaesthetic with a different chemical structure will reduce the risk of a second reaction.

> (i) m-NH_2-benzoic acid esters, e.g. proxymetacaine
> (ii) p-NH_2-benzoic acid esters, e.g. benoxinate
> (iii) benzoic acid amides, e.g. lignocaine
> (iv) unsubstituted benzoic acid esters, e.g. cocaine

When used as eye drops, anaesthetics in the first two classes have essentially identical characteristics in that they should produce adequate surface anaesthesia within 2 minutes and the effects should last 20 to 30 minutes. Eye drops containing unsubstituted benzoic acid esters or benzoic acid amides are generally used at high concentrations and are reserved for special cases where superficial surgery or substantial manipulation is to be performed. The patient should be told not to rub their eyes for at least 30 min after the use of the anaesthetics. Within 2 min, satisfactory anaesthesia should be present (and the patient will usually be able to indicate that this is so achieved) and various procedures can be undertaken for the next 10 to 15 min. If longer working periods are required, a higher concentration of the anesthetic (i.e. 1 % or 4 %) could be used initially (if available), or a second drop can be instilled a few minutes after the first. However, repeated instillations (i.e. more than 3 drops) within an hour or so must be considered as potentially toxic and a check should be made for any damage.

NOTE. Occasionally, following even routine use of anaesthetic or anaesthetic - fluorescein solutions, some stippling / punctate staining of the cornea can be seen. This may produce some acute discomfort, but should resolve readily within 24 h, especially with a little help from some preservative-free artificial tears (see Chapter 11). On rare occasions, very substantial and acute-onset stippling / glazing of the corneal surface can occur; this can be painful.! It is probably a form of hypersensitivity or allergic reaction but should resolve within 24 to 48 h, especially with the help of a few **Bayer**[R] **Aspirin** or **Anadin**[R] **All Night** (*p.o.*) as well as unpreserved artificial tears; a light eye patch may help but should only be used for 24 h.

Current UK-marketed topical ocular anaesthetic products include -

(**a**) proxymetacaine, also known as proparacaine. Is available as a 0.5 % ophthalmic solution in PoM **Minims**[R] **Proxymetacaine** (unit dose). Another product, PoM **Ophthaine**[R] (15 mL bottle) was discontinued in 1999. Proxymetacaine hydrochloride is a m-NH_2-benzoic acid ester. The Minims[R] product is best kept refrigerated. Proxymetacaine is unstable and can readily deteriorate if exposed to light even at room temperature.

A combination product, PoM **Minims**[R] **Proxymetacaine and fluorescein** contains proxymetacaine 0.5 % and fluorescein 0.25 %. This product should be refrigerated.

(**b**) benoxinate (also known as oxybuprocaine) is available as PoM **Minims**[R] **Benoxinate** which contains 0.4 % benoxinate. A 10 mL multi-use bottle (PoM **Dorsacaine**[R] **Eyedrops**) may also be available. Benoxinate is a p-NH_2-benzoic acid ester. The Minims[R] product should be kept cool but does not need refrigeration.

(**c**) amethocaine, also known as tetracaine. Is available as PoM **Minims**[R] **Amethocaine Hydrochloride** at both the 0.5 % and 1 % concentrations. A multi-use 10 mL bottle (PoM **Amethocaine Eye-drops** (generic) has also been available. Amethocaine hydrochloride is a p-NH_2-benzoic acid ester. The Minims[R] and multi-use bottle should be kept refrigerated. Once opened, the shelf-life of the multi-use bottle will be enhanced if kept refrigerated. Bottles for multi-use will likely contain anti-oxidants such as bisulphites.

(**d**) lignocaine (also known as lidocaine) it is available as PoM **Minims**[R] **Lignocaine and Fluorescein** at the 4 % concentration (with fluorescein 0.25 %). It is a benzoic acid amide used for situations where there are allergic reactions to the NH_2-benzoic acid esters (e.g. to the proxymetacaine - fluorescein combination or proxymetacaine alone), and for when longer anaesthesia is required or minor surgical intervention is required.

(**e**) cocaine. Cocaine is available as a controlled drug and only as CD **Cocaine Eye-Drops** (non-proprietary) at the 4 % concentration for use in special hospital clinics. These eye drops will only be prepared by specially licenced hospital pharmacies; a 5 or 10 mL bottle is usually prepared. Cocaine hydrochloride is an unsubstituted benzoic acid ester. Cocaine eye drops are not used for routine optometric practice, but by ophthalmologists for superficial surgery of the cornea. The commonest procedure is that for corneal epithelial debridement in cases of severe herpes simplex virus infections of the cornea. The anesthetic is so toxic that it "kills" the corneal cells and facilitates their removal. Cocaine is also a mydriatic as a result of an indirect adrenergic action (see Chapter 6).

(**f**) other local anaesthetics for ophthalmic use include bupivacaine, which is another benzoic acid amide. Bupivacaine and lignocaine (lidocaine for injection) are generally used by ophthalmologists as pre-surgical anaesthetics (for injection by the retrobulbar route) but can be injected into ocular tissue such as the eyelids. The injection procedure is known as infiltration and can be done with adrenaline (epinephrine) being present as well, to limit the passage of the anaesthetic into the circulation (where it can cause pronounced cardio-vascular effects). The surgical procedures include extra-ocular muscle surgery, to corneal transplants to cataract operations. These injectable anaesthetics are supplied in vials and are not used as eye drops. For bupivacaine, commercial products include PoM **Marcain**[R] at the 0.25 %, 0.5 % and 0.75 % concentrations or PoM **Marcain with adrenaline**[R] at the 0.25 % concentration with adrenaline (epinephrine) 1: 200,000 dilution. For lignocaine (lidocaine), commercial products include PoM **Lignocaine** (non-proprietary) at the 0.5 %, 1 % or 2 % concentration, and PoM **Xylocaine**[R] at the 0.5 %, 1 % or 2 % concentration with or without adrenaline (epinephrine) 1: 200,000. The inclusion of the epinephrine is to promote vasoconstriction around the injection site, and thus limit the diffusion of the anaesthetics into the peripheral vasculature (from where they could reach the heart without undergoing first pass metabolism). Another benzoic acid amide, ropivacaine (PoM **Naropin**[R]) has been recently introduced and has been used for ophthalmic surgery. It is considered to have less side effects than other related anaesthetics, and is available in a range of concentrations (0.2, 0.75 and 1 %).

AUTONOMIC PHARMACOLOGY of BODY AND EYE. I.

Purpose of chapter. Many of the actions of eyedrops, as well as drug-drug interactions, are determined by the activity of the autonomic nervous system. The principles of pharmacodynamics and pharmacokinetics can be used to define these actions by linking physiological actions and effects with specific drugs. In this chapter, only the mechanisms of those drugs that <u>directly</u> bind to receptors at nerve endplates to produce physiological actions will be covered.

In the autonomic nervous system (ANS), a general perspective is that some branches of the system are inhibited by the effects produced by stimulation of nerves in other branches. There is thus a net result for neural activities within peripheral nervous system (as opposed to the central nervous system; the CNS) and its is important that both aspects are considered, e.g. the sympathetic (adrenergic) system and the parasympathetic (cholinergic) branches of the ANS. The neural pathways of primary interest are those that originate in the CNS and move out to the periphery (i.e. *efferent* or out-flowing pathways) as opposed to pathways that start in the periphery and flow to the CNS (i.e. *afferent* or in-flowing sensory pathways).

The overall actions of sympathomimetic (adrenergic) drugs are generally opposite in action to the effects of parasympathetic (cholinergic) drugs. effects. Equally importantly, the overall actions of sympatholytic (adrenoceptor blocking) drugs are generally opposite to those of parasympatholytic (cholinoceptor blocking) drugs. For example, if a sympathetic drug speeds up the heart, a parasympathetic drug will usually slow down the heart. Equally well, while some adrenoceptor blocking drugs will slow down the heart, cholinoceptor blocking drugs will speed up the heart. For the eye, the pupil will dilate in response to sympathetic drugs and close in response to a parasympathetic drug, while it will close in response to some adrenoceptor blocking drugs and dilate in response to cholinoceptor blocking drugs. For each organ or tissue, there are subtle differences in the balances between the effects of sympathetic drugs and parasympathetic drugs simply because each organ has its own particular balance of sympathetic and parasympathetic innervation.

A. SITES RECEIVING SYMPATHETIC INNERVATION.

Two neurotransmitters produce sympathetic effects, these are epinephrine (adrenaline) and norepinephrine (noradrenaline). The first name is the currently accepted one, while the second name is the older British Approved Name (BAN). Both neurotransmitters are called catecholamines. The neurotransmitter released at nerve endings in muscles or glands is usually norepinephrine, while epinephrine circulates in our blood and in parts of the CNS to regulate blood flow to most tissues of the body.

Epinephrine, norepinephrine or *direct - acting adrenergic drugs* generally bind to adrenergic receptors to augment their function. This can however have opposite physiological consequences depending on whether the receptor is an excitatory type or an inhibitory type. Another way of stating this is that adrenergic drugs (including epinephrine) are able to act either as excitatory or inhibitory ligands at adrenergic receptors. Equally importantly, *direct - acting adrenoceptor blocking drugs* bind to adrenergic receptors to attenuate (block) the function of these receptors that would normally result from their interaction with either epinephrine or norepinephrine. This diversity means that a knowledge of the receptor type is very important in understanding adrenergic drug action; the following are clinically relevant -

(**a**) *alpha$_1$* receptors. These are most commonly found at peripheral (ANS) muscles, the vasculature and some glands; excitatory.

(**b**) *alpha$_2$* receptors. These are found at discrete sites in the CNS and some secretory sites, including some in the pancreas and the eye; inhibitory.

(**c**) *beta$_1$* receptors. These are found in select peripheral muscles, especially heart and bronchial system, and some sites in the vasculature; excitatory.

(**d**) *beta$_2$* receptors. These are principally found associated with select parts of the vasculature, especially that associated with secretory sites (including those of the tracheobronchial system and ciliary epithelium). They are also found associated with select smooth muscles such as those in the tracheobronchial system; generally inhibitory.

NOTE. A *beta$_3$* receptor, principally associated with the brochopulmonary system, the gastrointestinal (alimentary) tract, some endocrine glands and the CNS. No drugs are used at this time to specifically target this system.

EXAMPLES OF PHYSIOLOGICAL EFFECTS (**Table 1**). Epinephrine or phenylephrine [*fen-ill-ef-rin*] primarily act to increase the activity of excitatory adrenergic *alpha$_1$* receptors in the vasculature, and usually cause vasoconstriction and raise the blood pressure. Salbutamol [*sal-byoo-ta'mol*, e.g. PoM **Ventolin**^{R}] binds to adrenergic *beta$_2$* receptors in the tracheobronchial system to relax muscles and open up the airways. In contrast, clonidine [*kloe-ni-deen*, e.g. PoM **Catapres**^{R}] binds to adrenergic *alpha$_2$* receptors in the CNS and the vasculature. In the CNS, this clonidine binding augments the activity of inhibitory adrenergic pathways in the vasomotor centers of the brain stem. In the periphery, clonidine binding antagonises the normal vasoconstrictive action of epinephrine. With the combination of inhibitory CNS signals and peripheral antagonistic actions, vasodilation and decrease in blood pressure follow the administration of clonidine.

ADRENERGIC INNERVATION TO MAJOR SITES OF THE BODY
AND THE EXPECTED PHYSIOLOGICAL EFFECTS.

Items listed with a (?) indicate minimal clinical effect.

Table 1:

ORGAN	ADRENERGIC EFFECT	TYPE	ADRENERGIC BLOCKING
heart	pulse increased	$beta_1$	pulse decreased
heart A-V node	increased activity	$beta_1$	decreased activity
arterioles	dilate (usually)	$beta_2$	constriction (slight)
veins	constrict	$alpha_1$	dilation (slight)
airways	open	$beta_2$	close
airway secretions	decreased	alpha ? $beta_2$	increased ?
bladder	decreased emptying	$alpha_1$	increased emptying
pancreas acini	decreased secretion	$alpha_2$ $beta_2$	increased secretion
salivary glands	decreased secretion	$alpha_1$	increased secretion
sweat glands	increased secretion	$alpha_1$	decreased secretion
adrenal glands	increased secretion	$beta_1$	decreased secretion
EOM's	contraction	?	relaxation
lids (Mueller's)	lid elevation	$alpha_1$	(upper lid) close
lacrimal gland	increased secretion	beta ?	decreased secretion
conjunctiva	vasoconstriction	$alpha_1$	vasodilation
anterior uvea	vasodilation	$alpha_2$	no effect ?
iris dilator	contraction (open)	$alpha_1$	relaxation (close)
ciliary body	relaxation	$alpha_1$ beta	contraction ?
ciliary epithelium	decreased secretion (long term effect)	beta	decreased secretion

EXAMPLES: *Alpha*$_1$ adrenoceptor blocking drugs such as prazosin [*pra-zoe-sin*, PoM **Hypovase**^{R}] antagonise the normal vasoconstrictive effects of adrenaline on the vasculature, and produce vasodilatation and lower blood pressure. Such drugs have other uses too, e.g. to manage post-operative urinary retention (e.g. indoramin [*inn-dor-a'min*], PoM **Doralese**^{R}, or to promote regional peripheral vasodilatation to relieve Raynaud's syndrome (e.g. oral thymoxamine [*thye-mox-a'meen*], PoM **Opilon**^{R}). In contrast, *beta*$_1$ adrenoceptor blocking drugs such as metoprolol [*me-toe-proe'lole*, PoM **Lopresor**^{R}] block the normal stimulatory action of epinephrine on the heart and slow it down and, as secondary effect to slowing the pulse, lower the blood pressure. These examples are meant to show that there are a variety of adrenergic receptors that appear to be largely independent of each other in terms of their operation. Two different adrenergic receptors can be present within the same tissue or organ.

B. SITES RECEIVING PARASYMPATHETIC INNERVATION.

A single neurotransmitter is used, acetylcholine; it is not a catecholamine. The parasympathetic pathways use acetylcholine and the transmitter is also that present in many CNS pathways and at the ganglia linking the CNS with the ANS associated with the parasympathetic division. It is acceptable to divide these two roles (parasympathetic, versus CNS and ganglia), and to generalise on the receptor types.

Acetylcholine or *direct - acting cholinergic drugs* bind directly to cholinergic receptors to augment their function, and thus increase cholinergic synaptic activity. The pathways (or ganglia) can however be excitatory or inhibitory in nature depending on the end plate muscle or gland. *Direct-acting cholinoceptor blocking drugs* bind directly to cholinergic receptors to attenuate their function and thus counteract (or even reverse) the actions that would be produced by acetylcholine; most of these blocking drugs work in the peripheral ANS, rather than the CNS. Cholinoceptor blocking drugs are also known as "anticholinergics". The following receptor types operate with acetylcholine -

(**a**) nicotinic acetylcholine receptors located at discrete nerve bundles (nuclei) in the CNS and brain stem, and also at ganglia that serve both the sympathetic and parasympathetic branches of the ANS.

(**b**) muscarinic acetylcholine receptors located at discrete CNS nuclei, and at all end plates in the parasympathetic branch of the ANS.

EXAMPLES OF PHYSIOLOGICAL EFFECTS (**Table 2**). Acetylcholine binds to CNS receptors (nicotinic and muscarinic) to activate pathways that determine our state of awareness and motor (muscle) coordination.

Increased acetylcholine release at cardiac sites results in a slowing of the pulse, but increased CNS and peripheral parasympathetic activities generally improve muscle tone. Parasympathetic drugs have clinical uses to improve muscle function and increase both the motility of the alimentary tract and the function of the bladder.

CHOLINERGIC INNERVATION AT MAJOR SITES IN THE BODY
AND THE EFFECTS OF CLINICALLY USED DRUGS.

Items listed with a (?) indicate minimal clinical effect.

Table 2:

ORGAN	CHOLINERGIC EFFECT	BLOCKING EFFECT
heart S-A node	pulse slowed; vagal arrest	pulse increased
heart A-V node	decreased conduction AV block	increased conduction
atria	decreased contractility	shortened AP duration
arterioles	constriction	no effect ?
veins	dilation ?	constriction
intestine	increased motility	decreased motility
bladder	increased emptying	decreased emptying
airways	close; constriction	open
airway secretions	increase	decrease
pancreas acini	increased secretion	decreased secretion
salivary glands	increased secretion	decreased secretion
sweat glands	increased secretion	decreased secretion
adrenal glands	increased secretion	decreased secretion
eyelids	lid elevation	(upper lid) close
eyelids (orbicularis)	(reflex closing)	opening
conjunctival veins	dilation	constriction ?
anterior uvea veins	dilation	constriction
lacrimal acini	increased secretion	decreased secretion
iris sphincter	contraction (closing)	relaxation (opening)
ciliary body	contraction (myopia)	relaxation (cycloplegia)
ciliary epithelium	decreased secretion	no effect ?

EXAMPLES: Direct-acting cholinergic drugs such as pilocarpine [*pye-loh-kar-peen*, PoM **Salagen**[R]] bind to peripheral muscarinic receptors and produce parasympathetic effects such as increased salivation (as well as sweating and lacrimation) and can be used for this purpose. Other direct-acting cholinergics such as bethanechol [*bay-than-eh-kole*, PoM **Myotonine**[R]] are used to promote urinary output. Direct-acting cholinoceptor blockers such as atracurium [*aye-tra-cure-ee-um*, Pom **Tracrium**[R]] bind to nicotinic receptors, principally in ganglia, and block synaptic transmission to produce a general relaxation of all muscles, including those that permit us to breathe (diaphragm etc.) during major surgery. Cholinoceptor blocking drugs such as benztropine [*benz-troe-peen*, PoM **Cogentin**[R]] bind to select CNS-located muscarinic receptors in extra-pyramidal nuclei and produce a general sedating effect and reduction in uncontrolled motor activities. In addition, binding of benztropine to other sites in the CNS can alter our state of awareness such that hallucinations or similar effects develop.   Direct-acting cholinoceptor blockers such as atropine bind to muscarinic receptors at parasympathetic end plates in organs such as the heart (and increase the pulse) and the airways muscles (to improve airway function) and also produce general parasympatholytic effects such a dry mouth, reduced sweating, sensations of feeling hot / flushing, etc. Some of the atropine, at high doses, will enter the CNS and produce alterations in our state of awareness similar to benztropine. Other atropine-like drugs include hyoscine [*hye-oh-seen*, P **Buscopan**[R]] which is used to control GI tract upsets, ipratropium [*ee-pra-troe-pee-um*, PoM **Atrovent**[R]] which has selective effects on the airways, and others which are used for their selective actions on the bladder to control urinary incontinence, e.g. oxybutynin [*oxee-byoo-toe'nin*, PoM **Cystrin**[R]], tolterodine [*toll-tear-oh'deen*, PoM **Detrusitol**[R]] and propiverine [*pro-pi-ver'een*, PoM **Detrunorm**[R]]. For all the major parasympathetic sites, cholinergic and cholinergic blocking effects are summarised in the Table 2. What should be noted is that the cholinergic effects (Table 2) are generally opposite to those produced by the adrenergic system (Table 1).

C. SITES USING OTHER NEUROTRANSMITTERS

Autonomic pharmacology can be considered as involving only those physiological functions mediated by epinephrine and acetylcholine. While these two pathways unquestionably play a dominant and mutually-interactive role in the regulation of all bodily functions, there are also many drugs used in clinical medicine that can modulate or fine tune the sympathetic and parasympathetic systems. These drugs act at receptors using other neurotransmitters and can be viewed as ways of producing antagonistic effects to the sympathetic and parasympathetic pathways, especially in terms of their origins in the CNS. Despite the CNS-based action of many of these drugs, their use unquestionably has major effects in the peripheral organs and vasculature regulated by the autonomic nervous system. A small amount of knowledge of two of these secondary neurotransmitters, GABA and dopamine, is thus important for a clinical understanding of autonomic pharmacology.

(i) GABA (*gamma*-aminobutyric acid). GABA is a CNS and peripheral neurotransmitter found in both nerves and glial cells. It has a distinct role in regulating our state of awareness and its overall role is to modulate the excitatory pathways operated through norepinephrine or another catecholamine called serotonin (see Chapter 6). Hypoactivity in GABA - regulated pathways leads to states of over-reaction to stimulation and stress, and especially in our ability to relax and sleep. Drugs that are clinically used to directly bind to GABA receptors are called GABA-ergic drugs, and promote a more relaxed state because the neural hypoactivity is corrected and thus the over - reaction is attenuated. These drugs include *direct - acting GABA-ergics* that are classified as <u>benzodiazepines</u> (e.g. diazepam [*dye-ay-zee-pam*]; PoM **Valium**[R]) or <u>barbiturates</u> (e.g. amylobarbitone [*ay-meel-o-bar-bi-tone*]; also known as amobarbital; CD **Amytal**[R]). They are used to manage anxiety, and as pre-surgery sedatives and relaxants. They also have a wide use for insomnia (e.g. nitrazepam [*nye-traz-eh-pam*], PoM **Mogadon**[R]). Several types of GABAergic drugs are used as anti-epilepsy (anti-convulsant) drugs, e.g. clonazepam (PoM **Rivotril**[R]) and vigabatrin [*vye-gab-a'trin*] (PoM **Sabril**[R]). A GABA receptor blocker (antagonist) can be used to promote recovery of function in other types of motoneuron disorders, including those associated with stroke, e.g. baclofen [*bak'loe-fen*] (PoM **Lioresal**[R]).

Many GABAergic drugs can induce a very deep sleep or even a coma. Alcohol (ethyl alcohol) acts as a "CNS depressant" by boosting inhibitory GABA pathways. Depending on the individual, alcohol can produce uncontrolled or unpredictable mood swings before a general sedation develops. The initial phases reflect brain cortex mechanisms that promote relaxation and "release of our inhibitions". In high doses, alcohol can produce a stupor state. A mixture of alcohol with barbiturates can not only produce an acute-onset stupor state, but can even be fatal.

(ii) dopamine. Dopamine is another catecholamine that binds at many sites in the CNS where there are also norepinephrine - mediated synapses. Dopaminergic activity generally results in "activation" of inhibitory synapses which will antagonise the excitatory effects of norepinephrine. Alternatively, dopamine can furtehr "activate" adrenergic synapses that are already inhibitory (i.e. alpha$_2$ adrenergic pathways). In addition, dopamine - mediated synapses are also present at CNS and peripheral sites regulated by acetylcholine, and so dopamine regulates muscle coordination and can control tremors. Dopamine also regulates aspects of GI tract function.

Drugs in clinical use include *direct - acting dopaminergics* such as methyldopa [*me-theel-doe-pa*] (e.g. PoM **Aldomet**[R]) and levodopa [*lee-voe-doe-pa*] (e.g. in PoM **Sinemet**[R]). The first drug is primarily used to lower blood pressure because it antagonises the effects of the sympathetic system. The second drug, levodopa, is used to control fine motor tremors of

Parkinsonian' disease because it antagonises the uncontrolled actions of the CNS-parasympathetic system. There are also direct-acting dopaminergic blocking drugs (dopamine antagonists). The most important of these are lder drugs called neuroleptics (antipsychotics), which now recognised to have non-specific dopamine blocking actions, e.g. the phenothiazines used as major tranquillisers (chlorpromazine; *klor-proe'-ma-zeen*; PoM **Largactil**R). More specific dopamine blocking agents are now available, e.g. risperidone [*riss-pear-ee-done*] (PoM **Risperdal**R) and buspirone [*byoo-spye'rone*] (PoM **BusPar**R). Other dopaminergic blocking drugs have a CNS originating effect, but primarily affect the gastrointestinal (alimentary) tract, e.g. metoclopramide [*me-toe-cloe-prah-mide* (PoM **Gastromax**R) and domperidone (PoM **Motilum**R). These are used to indirectly augment the cholinergic regulation of GI tract motility (see earlier) by blocking CNS signals that stop the parasympathetic system functioning. They are used as anti-nausea agents (e.g. after strabismus surgery), and can also generally promote transit of food through the alimentary tract (upper-to-lower) when there is gastro-oesophageal spasm.

(**iii**) histamine. Histamine is another "neurotransmitter" found in most parts of the body. It is well known for its actions in allergic reactions but also serves as a CNS neurotransmitter, although its receptor pharmacology is not well understood. It is not a catecholamine but serves as a type of stimulant. CNS histamine receptor blockade produces the opposite effect (sedation, drowsiness etc.).

Certain histamine blocking drugs (e.g. hydroxyzine [*hye-droz'-i-zeen*]; PoM **Atarax**R) can be used to manage special types of anxiety because of their sedating effects. Other select-acting histamine blocking drugs can be used as sleep aids (e.g. promazine [*proe'ma-zeen*], PoM **Sominex**R; diphenhydramine [*dye-fen-hye'dra-meen*], P **Nytol**R). Antihistamines can be used to control allergies and a well-known ADR associated with the use of higher doses of other older "sedating" anti-histamines (e.g. chlorpheniramine, P **Piriton**R) is drowsiness, which can significantly impair a persons ability to perform tasks such as driving or operating heavy machinery. Lastly, other CNS-acting histamine receptor blocking drugs can be used to manage migraine or nausea (e.g. cyclizine [*sye'kli-zeen*]; PoM **Migril**R, PoM **Valoid**R), because of their sedative / calming effects.

AUTONOMIC PHARMACOLOGY of BODY and EYE. II

Purpose of chapter. In chapter 5, the effects of direct-acting drugs on various bodily functions, and the eye, were covered. Such drugs bind directly to receptors and either directly mimic, augment or block the response that would be produced by the binding of a neurotransmitter to those receptors. Such direct-acting drugs will produce their effects until they are metabolised and eliminated, and then the physiological functions return to being regulated only by the natural neurotransmitters. However, there are a large number of drugs that work indirectly in that they change the way in which the neurotransmitters are released or metabolised. The end result is similar in that physiological functions are increased or decreased but the mechanism of achieving this is indirect and thus usually has a different time base of action than direct-acting drugs (i.e. very short or very long duration); this provides an important clinical option for medication. The mechanisms by which such indirect actions of drugs can be produced will be addressed in this chapter, along with clinical examples. The clinical use of one of these drugs (botulinum toxin) will also be covered in detail.

To understand indirect actions of autonomic drugs, the mechanisms underlying the synthesis, release and biotransformation of neurotransmitters have to be understood. For nerve-nerve, nerve-muscle or nerve-gland transmission, there are two components; the pre- and post-synaptic cells. The process of junctional transmission is initiated by the arrival of an action potential (or sequence of action potentials) at the pre-junctional cells. The resultant changes in electrical potential difference that occur within the pre-synaptic axon cell then promote the release of an excitatory or an inhibitory neurotransmitter chemical from vesicles in the terminal into the synapse (the synaptic cleft). The synthesis and storage of the neurotransmitters and a specific mechanism for release of the neurotransmitters is essential for release of neurotransmitters to occur in response to the electrical changes. Once released, the neurotransmitters diffuse across the synaptic cleft and can then interact with receptors on the post - synaptic membrane. The neurotransmitters will then either be re-absorbed back into the nerve terminals and / or biotransformed to an inactive metabolite that diffuses away. The processes of synthesis, release and biotransformation, and their modulation by drugs (medicines) will be considered in this chapter.

1. ADRENERGIC NEUROTRANSMISSION.

Norepinephrine is synthesized in nerves and nerve terminals from the catecholamine dopamine, by an enzyme called dopamine hydroxylase. This noradrenaline can be stored in vesicles in pre-synaptic terminals. Some of the norepinephrine will however be used for the synthesis of epinephrine using an enzyme called N-methyltransferase. The resultant epinephrine can also be stored in pre-synaptic terminals. The storage process involves a specific mechanism and if this storage does not occur, these neurotransmitters will either simply be released after being synthesized or be inactivated (see later). In response to electrical stimulation, the neurotransmitters can be released. After binding to their different receptors, both these neurotransmitters will dissociate from the receptors and be re-absorbed (re-uptake) back into the pre-synaptic terminals. After re-uptake, these catecholamine neurotransmitters are inactivated by catechol-O-methyltransferase (abbreviated COMT) or monoamine oxidase (abbreviated MAO) enzymes in the pre-synaptic terminal. There are two types of monoamine oxidase, type A and type B, depending on where the nerve terminals are in the body. There are several ways in which the overall process can be *indirectly* modified by drugs -

(**i**) the storage of catecholamines is blocked by guanethidine [*gwahn-eth-i-deen*] (e.g. oral PoM **Ismelin**R) and, as a result, pre-synaptic terminals are slowly depleted of catecholamines. In the short term, the extra release of neurotransmitter may produce sympathetic effects but the main effect is that in the long term, where the progressive release will eventually lead to an indirect blockade of neurotransmission because the nerve terminals are depleted. This overall indirect adrenergic-blocking (or neurone blocking) effect produces peripheral vasodilatation and lowered blood pressure.

(**ii**) the release of catecholamines from pre-synaptic terminals can be non-specifically increased, independent of action potentials, by cocaine. This results in an overall uncontrolled sympathetic effect that results in agitation, elevated blood pressure, tachycardia ("racing of the heart"), dilated pupils, and hyperflexia or convulsions. These effects accompany the use of the drug as a hallucinogen, and coma may also develop following abuse of this controlled drug (PoMCD). In the short term, cocaine acts as an indirect adrenoceptor stimulant (since it produces extra release of epinephrine and norepinephrine to bind to receptors). In the long term however, this uncontrolled release can result in selective blockade of neurotransmission because terminals are depleted; both effects are indirect. There are also other *select indirect - acting adrenergics* that act in the CNS (e.g. amphetamines, dexamphetamine [*dex-am-fet-a-meen*; e.g. PoMCD **Dexedrine**R) and methylphenidate [*meth-ill-fen'i-date*]; oral PoMCD **Ritalin**R); they have legitimate uses in ADD (attention deficit disorder; also known as attention deficit hyperactivity disorder, ADHD) and drug-induced problems with staying awake (narcolepsy). These drugs produce a mild sympathomimetic CNS "high" with peripheral effects, both because of their neuro-transmitter-releasing effects on adrenergic synapses, and on receptors for another catecholamine, serotonin (see below).

(**iii**) the re-uptake of catecholamines back into the pre-synaptic terminals can be blocked by a group of drugs known as "tricyclic anti-depressants", with some drugs actually being tetracyclics. All of the drugs have indirect-acting adrenergic effects, but for each drug the re-uptake of one catecholamine may be blocked more than others. There are now several groups of drugs in this category that include drugs labelled as NARI's ("noradrenaline re-uptake inhibitor), SNRI's ("serotonin-noradrenaline re-uptake inhibitors") and NASSA's ("noradrenaline and specific serotonergic antidepressants"), in addition to the 'tricyclics'. For example, norepinephrine re-uptake is primarily affected by the tetracyclic maprotiline [*ma-proe-ti-leen*; oral PoM **Ludiomil**^R), and same probably also applies to mianserin [*mee-an-sir'in*], another tetracyclic. Reboxetine (PoM **Edronax**^R) is a newer drug and is considered so selective that it has been labelled as a NARI. For others, the mechanisms are more complex. While the metabolite of a tricyclic antidepressant called clomipramine [*kloe-mi-pra-meen*; oral PoM **Anafranil**^R) is considered to block norepinephrine re-uptake, clomipramine itself blocks serotonin re-uptake; this is a unique pro-drug effect. Other newer drugs are considered to block re-uptake of serotonin much more than norepinephrine; these drugs were thus labelled as SNRI's, e.g. venlafaxine [*ven-lah-fax-een*; oral PoM **Efexor**^R]. Another new group of drugs are considered to block norepinephrine re-uptake to a similar extent to serotonin re-uptake, and have been labelled as NaSSA's, e.g. mirtazapine; PoM **Zispin**^R). Some of these drugs are less specific since these tricyclics not only generally affect norepinephrine and serotonin re-uptake at the same time, but also can have pronounced anti-muscarinic (cholinergic blocking) actions, e.g. amitriptyline ([*a-mee-trip'ti-leen*], PoM **Tryptizol**^R) or trimipramine ([*try-mi-prah-meen*], oral PoM **Surmontil**^R). They can used to promote sedation in depressed patients (e.g. amitriptyline), or as sleep aids in depressed patients (trimipramine).

(**iv**) the biotransformation of catecholamines, after re-uptake, by monoamine oxidase can be inhibited by MAO inhibitors such as phenelzine [*fenn-ell-zeen*] (e.g. oral PoM **Nardil**^R). If the inactivation of norepinephrine or epinephrine is reduced, then a general sympathetic effect is produced; the drug-mediated effect is indirect because the actual adrenergic receptors are not affected. The dose of phenelzine should be carefully controlled to limit the extent of these effects throughout the body. The use of phenelzine is designed to boost brain catecholamine levels and thus provide a mood-elevating effect; these MAO inhibitors are thus used as anti-depressants. Phenelzine is a non-specific MAO inhibitor since it will inhibit both type A and type B forms of the enzyme. However, other indirect-acting sympathomimetics are specific inhibitors of MAO type A (e.g. moclobemide [*mo'kloe-be'mide*]; oral PoM **Manerix**^R) which is used as an anti-depressant and known as a "reversible inhibitor of monoamine oxidase type A", a RIMA. There is also an inhibitor of MAO type B (e.g. selegiline [*sell-edge-ee-leen*]; oral PoM **Eldepryl**^R) used to manage Parkinsonian disease); selegiline also preferentially blocks the inactivation of the catecholamine dopamine, as well as norepinephrine and epinephrine.

2. SEROTONINERGIC NEUROTRANSMISSION.

Serotonin is another amine neurotransmitter that principally acts in the CNS. Serotonin is the same as 5-hydroxytryptamine and 5-HT (an accepted abbreviation). Serotonin is considered to act at various excitatory nerve - nerve synapses in the CNS and brain and thus has some actions that are similar to epinephrine and norepinephrine. In addition, portions of the cerebral vasculature (especially the Circle of Willis) are considered to be very sensitive to serotonin; differences in serotonin levels are thought to determine the relative intra-cranial blood flow or localized stasis in blood flow compared to the extra-cranial blood vessels. Serotonin - modulating drugs can thus have both mood - elevating effects and vasoactive properties.

Serotonin (5-HT) is synthesised by the action of the enzyme aromatic amino acid decarboxylase present in nerves cells and glial cells. The neuro-transmitter is stored in vesicles and released in response to pre-synaptic electrical potential changes. Once released, serotonin can bind to at least three different receptor types known as $5-HT_1$, $5-HT_2$, $5-HT_3$, $5-HT_4$ etc receptors (that have a number of sub-types as well). The receptor specificity (selectivity) for clinically - used serotoninergic drugs is still poorly defined, and opinions on the selectivity are widely debated. After dissociating from its receptors, serotonin is re-absorbed into the pre-synaptic terminals by a specific re-uptake mechanism. This re-uptake terminates the serotoninergic neurotransmission and some of serotonin will be biotransformed by monoamine oxidase. There are three types of drugs used to modulate serotoninergic neurotransmission -

(i) sumatriptan [*soo-mah-trip-tan*] (oral PoM **Imigran**[R]) and related drugs principally bind to $5-HT_1$ receptors (as $5-HT_1$ agonists) to promote cerebral blood flow (as a result of a vasoconstrictive action) and relieve migraine attacks. Sumatriptan is also available as a self-administered subcutaneous injection *(s.c.)*, and as a nasal spray.

(ii) hallucinogenic drugs, such as LSD, bind to a poorly defined sub-group of $5-HT_1$ receptors to produce a CNS "high" (in addition to the vasoconstriction and increased cerebral blood flow).

(iii) *indirect-acting serotoninergic, or* serotonin-stimulating drugs are very widely used as mood-elevators and anti-depressants. These include fluoxetine [*floo-ox-e' teen*] (e.g. oral PoM **Prozac**[R]), and sertraline [*sir-tra-leen*] (e.g. oral PoM **Lustral**[R]). These drugs are labelled as serotonin re - uptake inhibitors (SRI's) or selective serotonin re-uptake inhibitors (SSRI's).

3. CHOLINERGIC NEUROTRANSMISSION.

Acetylcholine is synthesised by an enzyme called choline acetyltransferase (ChAT) that is present in the pre-junctional axon and nerve cell bodies. After synthesis, the acetylcholine is stored in vesicles in the pre - synaptic terminal. An action potential causes release of acetylcholine by exocytosis. After release, the acetylcholine can bind to post-junctional receptors and then is inactivated by acetylcholinesterase or cholinesterase enzymes. There are several ways in which this overall process can be indirectly modified -

(i) The release (exocytosis) of the acetylcholine can be blocked by botulinum toxin A. If the release of acetylcholine is blocked, an indirect blockade of neurotransmission occurs. If generally affecting the body, as in food poisoning caused by this toxin (botulism), severe cholinergic blocking effects occur and require administration of botulism anti-toxin (available from poison control centres). High doses can cause general paralysis and even death. This effect can however be used to advantage to locally paralyse specific muscles (see section below).

(ii) the biotransformation of the acetylcholine by acetylcholine esterase (abbreviated AcChE or AChE; but not ACE) or choline esterase (ChE) can be inhibited by acetylcholinesterase inhibitors, also known as anti-cholinesterases. These *indirect-acting cholinergic drugs* do not bind to the cholinergic receptor but instead decrease the rate of biotransformation of AcCh; they do this by reversibly or irreversibly inhibiting AcChE and/ or ChE. As a result, synaptic levels of AcCh are maintained at a higher levels for a longer period of time, with a resultant augmentation of the parasympathetic synapse. Examples include neostigmine, donepezil, edrophonium, and parathion. Neostigmine [*nee-oh-stig-meen*; e.g. oral PoM **Prostigmin**[R]] is a short-acting and reversible AcChE inhibitor that is used to improve muscle tone in such conditions as myasthenia gravis, or to correct urinary retention post-operatively. Donepezil [*donn-ep-ee-zil*; PoM **Aricept**[R]] is an example of a CNS-selective AcChE inhibitor and has been introduced as a potential therapy for senile dementia's such as Alzheimers disease. Edrophonium [*ed-roe-foe-nee-um*] (e.g. as once marketed as PoM **Camsilon**[R] or **Tensilon**[R]) is an ultra-short acting, reversible AcChE inhibitor also used to temporarily improve muscle tone, but also as an *i.v.* or *i.m.* injection as a test for myasthenia gravis. It would likely only be encountered in a specialist hospital clinic [as **Edrophonium chloride** (generic), or be prepared by the hospital pharmacy]. Other anti-cholinesterases include chemicals used as pediculocides for head and pubic lice (e.g. malathion [*ma'la-thye-on*]; P **Prioderm**[R]) and these are classified as very long-lasting and irreversible since they bind to acetylcholinesterase and cholinesterase with very high affinity and remain bound for many days; severe parasympathetic adverse effects can result in death following accidental exposure because of the irreversible action.

CLINICAL USE OF BOTULINUM A TOXIN FOR THE EYE.

Special pharmaceuticals are available (e.g. PoM **Dysport**[R], PoM **Botox**[R]) that is a sterile solution of a botulinum A toxin - haemagglutinin complex. The haemagglutinin part of the complex is because the toxin (extracted from *Clostridium botulinum*) is composed of a protein which is the toxin and two other proteins with haemagglutinating activity. The extracted toxin is actually dried (by a process called freeze-drying) and sold in a sealed vial that must be kept frozen. Shortly before use, this lyophilised powder has to be dissolved in a sterile saline. The concentration of the toxin is measured in something called a unit, rather than as g/ 100 mL or mg/mL etc. This unit of activity is equivalent to the LD_{50} for mice, and is an incredibly small quantity (i.e. about 0.25 ng). While botulinum toxins can be lethal, the LD_{50} for man is at least 500 X higher.

Injections of botulinum A toxin are indicated for treatment of three main types of neuromuscular disorders where the disorder is characterized by the over-activity (contraction) of an easily defined muscle group. These disorders include essential blepharospasm, hemifacial spasm (the two main indications) and also select cases of strabismus (squint), including those associated with 3rd or 6th nerve palsies after trauma.

The treatment of strabismus is outlined below but similar principles apply to the treatment of the other two conditions. In select cases of horizontal strabismus involving the medial and lateral rectus muscles and where there is usually no more than 40 prism dioptres of deviation, the treatment involves injection of the toxin solution (0.1 to 0.25 mL) into the muscle that is responsible for the eso- or exo-deviation. The treatment tends to be more successful for esophorias. The actual doses of toxin are usually 2.5 to 5 units, unless the procedure is performed on infants less than 2 years of age where only 1 to 2 units are used. The goal of the injection is to infiltrate the muscle tissue with toxin solution, especially around the nerve-muscle junctions, to produce what is termed chemical denervation. This is achieved because the toxin is rapidly taken up by the pre-synaptic nerve terminals and binds to the acetylcholine-storage vesicles. As a result of this binding, the normal release of acetylcholine is totally blocked and the nerve-muscle endplates degenerate, producing a total paralysis of the affected muscle bundles. To achieve maximum effects, the toxin needs to be injected into the sites with the highest density of active endplates. This is achieved as follows. The ocular surface is anaesthetised with one or two drops of amethocaine 1 % or proxymetacaine 0.5 % eye drops (see chapter 4), although infants may also be sedated / anaesthetised with *i.m.* ketamine (e.g. PoM **Ketalar**[R]; 0.5 to 1 mg / kg body weight). A topical decongestant (vasoconstrictor) or subconjunctival injection (of dilute epinephrine) may be used to help visualize the insertion of the rectus muscles. The eye is first turned to expose the anterior insertion point of the muscle that is to be injected and a very fine needle-electrode (27 to 30 gauge) is carefully inserted. The eye is then turned back to a normal position or even to the opposite deviation and the needle slowly pushed in. The needle-electrode is connected to an amplifier that emits a tone and, with another electrode placed on the patients' forehead, the electrical signals generated by the muscle (an electromyograph or EMG) can be heard. As the muscle is stretched as the eye is moved to the normal or adductive position and the needle-electrode reaches a position about 2.5 mm posterior to the original insertion, the EMG frequency should be at its highest level and the toxin can be injected safely into the muscle. If the needle-electrode passes the maximum density of end-plates or even goes through the muscle, the EMG frequency tone goes down substantially. The eye is usually lightly patched / padded for a few hours after the injections. Some recommend that the patient sit upright for 4 hours after the injections and limit physical activity to limit toxin spread into adjacent tissue. Paralysis occurs in 3 to 6 days.

The needle-electrode is essential for safe and effective delivery of the toxin. Toxin injection into the connective tissue outside of the muscle can result in its leakage into other muscles or, in the extreme, result in the perforation of the globe. The needle-electrode also should not perforate blood vessels. As a precaution to check that the needle did not penetrate the globe, the pupil is usually dilated after the injection and indirect ophthalmoscopy carried out to check for internal haemorrhage or other signs of perforation. If the botulinum A toxin injection is successful, deviations of 40 prism dioptres can be reduced by 75 % or more. The goal is to produce an ocular alignment that is within 5 to 10 prism dioptres of normal orthophoria; over-correction (e.g. changing an esophoria into an exophoria) is a rare complication of the procedure and at least 1/3 of cases will be under-corrected with the first injection so it may be repeated several months later. The residual phoria can be corrected with spectacles.

The chemo-denervation produces paralysis of the injected muscle (and it should be noted that botulinum toxin is really the only ophthalmic drug that paralyses muscles, as opposed to relaxing them) but the effect is not permanent. Over a period of several weeks to several months, the nerve-endplates regrow (or "re-sprout") around the injection site to restore muscle action. However, it is hoped that the regrowth will be at a level which is compatible with the new position of the eye and the required muscle tension and innervational balance to now produce coordinated and yoked eye movements (as opposed to a full regrowth that could again turn the eye). The success of the procedure is thus real only known sometime after the injection when the effects of the toxin have abated. The first true assessments of eye alignment can be made when reasonable ocular motility is restored to all other muscles (excluding side effects; see below) and this is usually at the 6 to 8 week time point. The full assessment of success will be made 6 to 9 months later when the toxin effects have completely gone and neurological yoking had been fully restored. For mobile eyes, the procedure can mean a change in phorias (including those for intermittent tropias) down to a level manageable with spectacles and the difference between limited convergence with diplopia to easily accomplished convergence (up to normal near points for the patients age) without diplopia. In some cases however, the procedure produces under-correction and the induced deviation declines with time. The procedure can be repeated, providing the muscle tissue was not damaged by the first set of injections. The toxin injections are rarely effective for patients who have previously had strabismus surgery simply because the resultant scar tissue allows for diffusion of the toxin into adjacent sites and produces side effects.

Some other complications can develop if the toxin enters other muscles. A ptosis can develop or, in rare cases, pupil dilation (iris sphincter paralysis) or reduce accommodation (ciliary muscle paralysis). A temporary but mild ptosis is a fairly common side effect but disappears by the time of the first full assessment at 5 to 7 weeks. Perforation or haemorrhaging (or both) is likely to accompany any effects on the intraocular muscles; the needle does not have to obviously enter (puncture) the globe for the toxin to leak in.

4. SITES RECEIVING GABAergic INNERVATION

GABA is synthesised in nerve terminals and released in response to electrical stimulation. After release, it is inactivated by GABA transaminase. An indirect-acting GABAergic drug can either augment GABA-mediated transmission by promoting GABA release (e.g. sodium valproate; PoM **Convulex**[R]) while other GABAergics have direct and some indirect-action through GABA transaminase so enhancing GABA levels in the synapses (e.g. vigabatrin, PoM **Sabril**[R]; gabapentin, PoM **Neurontin**[R]).

5. SITES RECEIVING DOPAMINERGIC TRANSMISSION

Dopamine is synthesised in nerve terminals from tyrosine. Actually, a specific precursor of dopamine is synthesised (called L-DOPA), which is then biotransformed in the body into dopamine. The dopamine is then released, acts at its receptors, generally undergoes re-uptake and is then inactivated by biotransformation (by dopamine decarboxylase, monoamine oxidase-B and catechol-O-methyl transferase, COMT). In the clinical use of dopamine to manage Parkinson's, oral levodopa is actually biotransformed into dopamine in the body and an inhibitor of dopamine decarboxylase (a drug called carbidopa) is often co-administered with levodopa (e.g. PoM **Sinemet**[R]) to boost dopamine levels. A second approach to boost dopamine levels is to use drugs that inhibit monoamine oxidase-B (e.g. selegiline, PoM **Eldepryl**[R]). A new approach is to use COMT inhibitors, e.g. tolcapone (e.g. was PoM **Tasmar**[R]) and entacapone (PoM **Comtess**[R]) but there have been some serious ADR's with this last group of drugs.

MYDRIATIC OPTHALMIC SOLUTIONS AND USES

Purpose of chapter. Mydriatics are commonly used to facilitate an examination of the inside of the eye. The goal of the use of a mydriatic drug is to produce a relative dilation of the pupil from that pupil diameter that would be adopted under moderate-to-high intensity illumination. Several different drugs or drug combinations can however be used to achieve this effect. The mechanism of action of these drugs, their expected clinical effects and details of their actual use will be covered in this chapter.

When using mydriatics, a single drop of mydriatic can be instilled into the eye and mydriasis could be complete within 20 to 30 min. This is therefore a single, pulse-delivery of drug. In some cases however, more than one drop will be indicated to either achieve a reasonable pupil dilation and / or to produce a dilation that shows better resistance to light stimuli. In such cases, the second or third drops should be instilled with at least one minute between them, and preferably at 3 to 5 minute intervals. This is a multiple pulse delivery of the mydriatic drug to the iris tissue.

MECHANISMS OF ACTION OF MYDRIATICS

Mydriatic eyedrops can dilate the pupil via one of two mechanisms, or both mechanisms can be used. If an *alpha*$_1$-adrenergic drug is used, the dilator muscle will contract and the pupil opens slowly; the dilated pupil retains some of its light sensitivity so will still constrict under bright light. If a cholinergic blocking drug is used, the sphincter muscle will relax and the pupil opens faster; the dilated pupil should loose its light sensitivity.

GENERAL GUIDELINES FOR USE OF MYDRIATICS

No pharmaceutical should be used on the eye when there is a known hypersensitivity to the drug, or any of the other ingredients of the pharmaceutical (e.g. the preservatives, buffers, stabilisers etc.); this rule is particularly applicable to some mydriatics.

The use of a mydriatic is contraindicated, *in routine optometric practice*, in -

(a) cases of known narrow angle glaucoma (i.e. a sub-acute or chronic condition, or a history suggestive of the same) associated with a physical reduction (impairment) of outflow facility.

(b) cases with narrow angles, i.e. in eyes that, on the basis of physical assessment, have an angle that by Van Herrick criteria are likely to close under the action of a mydriatic. These would be grade I (or 1: 1/4) angles or those that appear closed (grade 0) despite lack of associated signs and symptoms.

(**c**) in cases of obvious dislocation (subluxation) of the crystalline lens, or an IOL (intra-ocular lens). While in most cases, the lens or IOL will move posteriorly and not create any acute problems, there is always the chance that the lens or IOL will tilt or completely dislocate anteriorly to give endothelial contact and corneal oedema. Such pupil dilations should be done in a hospital setting.

(**d**) in eyes where an iris-supported /iris-clipped, iris-sutured or iris-stapled IOL is in place. Pupillary dilation may simply dislocate or de-center the lens because it is relatively easy to dilate a pupil eccentrically, or (in the extreme) tear or rip the iris tissue leading to acute iritis and possible precipitation of 2° glaucoma.

The use of any mydriatic should be *approached with caution* when there is-

(**e**) the presence or possibility of a systemic medication-related pupil effect, although this is NOT to say that the use of the mydriatic is contraindicated (even if you might read some sources or articles that categorically state that mydriatics should not be used when a patient is on a certain medication etc.). A history- and ocular health-orientated judgement should then be made as to whether the addition of the mydriatic to the patient (as eye drops) will leave them significantly at risk for ocular complications (e.g. angle closure) or systemic problems (e.g. hypertension). The key points to consider here are (i) the actual dose of the medications that the patient is taking, (ii) how they are responding to the medication(s), (iii) whether there are any ocular effects. If uncertain whether to proceed, the physician prescribing the systemic drugs should be consulted. A similar consultation could also be made prior to dilating a patient with any really serious systemic illness.

SPECIFIC MYDRIATIC EYEDROPS

A. tropicamide [*troe-pick-a'-mide*] eye-drops are indicated for routine mydriasis. Eye drops containing tropicamide are probably not only the first-choice mydriatic, but the most commonly used ones.

(**i**) commercial products- PoM **Minims**[R] **Tropicamide** Eye-drops in single-use containers. The containers are stamped TRO 0.5 or 1.0. Multi-use bottles of tropicamide 0.5 % and 1.0 % are also marketed (PoM **Mydriacyl**[R], 5 mL bottles).Tropicamide was also available as PoM **NODS**[R] **Tropicamide** Ophthalmic applicator strips, with the single 125 microgram NODS strip impregnated with the equivalent of 1 drop of tropicamide 1 % solution; the product was discontinued in May, 1996.

(**ii**) ingredients of the eye drops are tropicamide 0.5 or 1 %. The nature of the vehicle is such that the eye drops may produce a marked stinging sensation. The eye drops are non-preserved. Products should NOT be refrigerated but should be stored in a cool dark place.

(iii) indicated for use as a routine mydriatic to facilitate any aspect of intra-ocular examination. The pupil loses much of its light sensitivity as the dilation develops and thus does not shut down much in most patients under slit lamp or ophthalmoscopy illumination etc.

(iv) contraindications (C/I) specific for the use of tropicamide eye drops. There are no listed contraindications (e.g. systemic medications etc.) other than a known sensitivity to the drug or the pharmaceutical.

(v) specific precautions (S/P) approach for tropicamide eye drops if patient is taking any medication that has resulted in a slightly dilated pupil, e.g. direct or indirect acting sympathomimetics (MAO inhibitors, SNRI's, NARI's, tricyclic antidepressants) or other cholinergic blocking drugs (e.g. homatropine, hyoscine [scopolamine]). In such cases, the apparent effects of the tropicamide eye drops may be prolonged.

(vi) pharmacokinetics of tropicamide eye drops. A single drop of tropicamide 0.5 % should produce 2 to 3 mm dilation within 20 minutes. The rate and magnitude of the dilation can be expected to increase either by using the 1 % concentration or increasing the number of drops. Pupil recovery can be within 2 to 3 h following use of just 1 *gtt* 0.5 %, but longer with larger doses, up to 18 h may be required for full recovery.

(vii) effect of patient age on pharmacokinetics of tropicamide: older patients tend to dilate less well. The actual magnitude of the mydriasis may well be similar in older (over 60 yrs) *vs.* younger patients, but since there is often an age-dependent decrease in resting pupil size, the overall efficacy of tropicamide can be expected to be less in older patients; two or even three drops could indicated in senior patients to ensure adequate dilation.

(viii) effect of ocular pigmentation on pharmacokinetics of tropicamide eye drops: very dark pigment may reduce efficacy - controversial !. Some have stated that the mydriatic effect of tropicamide is independent of iris color; others not only suggest but document that the response is smaller in patients with darker eyes, and *vice versa*. To be on the safe side, assume that the darker the pigmentation, the more resistant the pupil will be to dilate and increase the dosage accordingly.

NOTE. There is limited evidence to suggest that some other factor, possibly genetic, plays a role in determining the mydriatic response to tropicamide such that some individuals with darker irides may show a greater dilation than those with blue irides !.

B. phenylephrine [*fen-ill-ef'rin*] is not generally indicated for use on its own in the optometric office, either as a 2.5 % or 10 % solution; the latter is more likely used by an ophthalmologist, as a pre-surgical mydriatic.

The reason for the limited utility of phenylephrine, as a mydriatic on its own for general optometric practice, simply relates to expected efficacy.

(i) <u>Commercial products</u>. **Minims**[R] **Phenylephrine hydrochloride** eye-drops containing either 2.5 % or 10 % phenylephrine. The **Minims**[R] **Phenylephrine** 2.5 % is actually classified as a P Medicine, but should never be available to the public-at-large. The packs are stamped PHE 2.5 or PHE 10. A 10 % solution is also available as **Phenylephrine Eyedrops** (generic) in a 10 mL multi-use bottle.

(ii) <u>ingredients</u>- phenylephrine HCl 2.5 % or 10 %. The **Minims**[R] is preservative-free but may contain the stabiliser sodium <u>metabisulphite</u>, an anti-oxidant, which a patient may be allergic to. Metabisulphites would be expected for the multi-use bottles. Phenylephrine products should be stored in a cool place and away from light both before and after opening. Different manufacturers have provide different instructions on storage; they should not be frozen. The eye drops have a pink or straw colour when degraded.

(iii) <u>indications for use</u> as a mydriatic. Phenylephrine is rarely used on its own in optometric practice because lower concentrations of the drug are generally used (i.e 2.5 %). Its principal application is in combination mydriatics (e.g. phenylephrine with tropicamide; see below).The reason for its infrequent use is that, even with a pupil dilation of 3 mm (see below), the pupil still retails moderate or full light sensitivity. As a result, while the pupil may stay dilated long enough during photographic flash procedures as for fundus photography or with very brief ophthalmoscopic examination, it will certainly constrict to unusable levels with binocular indirect ophthalmoscopy, etc., (i.e. to less than 6 mm diameter).

 (iv) <u>contraindications</u> (**C/I**) specific for use of phenylephrine eye drops. These include known cardiac disorders, marked systemic hypertension (i.e. > 150/90 blood pressure), any history of aneurysms/ stroke, concurrent usage of any medications for cardiac arrhythmias or high blood pressure that would predispose the patient to a significant systemic response from the unavoidable systemic absorption of the eye drops, i.e. even eye drops are capable of raising blood pressure. The most important group of medications here are those that are used to maintain a low blood pressure in patients with chronic (arterial) disease, since it is in such patients that the "pressor" effect of the phenylephrine eye drops could be most marked. The group of drugs to be mainly considered here are the CNS-acting adrenergic agonists, and drugs that have some effects on these special pathways, e.g. oral clonidine (e.g. PoM **Catapres**[R]), oral bethanidine (PoM **Bethanidine**[R], generic), oral guanethidine(e.g. PoM **Ismelin**[R]), and oral methyldopa (PoM **Aldomet**[R]).

(v) <u>specific precautions</u> (**S/P**) (**INT**) approach for phenylephrine eye drops in any patient taking direct- or indirect-acting sympathomimetic drugs at dosages that may predispose them to a systemic sympathetic response.

These drugs include the MAO inhibitors (e.g. phenelzine, PoM **Nardil**[R]), the tricyclic anti-depressants (e.g. trimipramine, PoM **Surmontil**[R]), NARI's (e.g. oral reboxetine, PoM **Edronax**[R]), SNRI's (e.g. oral venlafaxine, PoM **Efexor**[R]), NaSSA's (e.g.mirtazapine, PoM **Zispin**[R]) and SSRI's (e.g. oral fluoxetine, PoM **Prozac**[R]). Similarly, the use of phenylephrine eye drops should be approached with cation in patients taking sympatholytic drugs of the *beta*-blocking type used for blood pressure control, e.g. metoprolol (PoM **Lopresor**[R]). The 'pressor' response may produce unwanted fluctuations in blood pressure. **(S/P)** The use of phenylephrine 10 % eye drops in elderly patients is more likely to cause pigment release from the iris tissue, as compared to the 2.5 % solution. The of mydriatics should be approached with caution in patients with open angle (simple) glaucoma; the use of adrenergic mydriatics is not contraindicated, regardless of a patients' anti-glaucoma medications (unless the patient also has systemic diseases listed as C/I for phenylephrine).

(**vi**) pharmacokinetics for phenylephrine eye drops. With a single drop of the 2.5 % solution, pupil dilation can be expected to take 50 to 60 min, but is usually incomplete. Some individuals will not dilate well, and the average dilation is only around 2 mm. A period of 12 to 24 h is required for full recovery. With two drops, the time to dilation may be only 45 min but the net dilation may increase to 3 mm and the pupil can be expected to show lesser closure on illumination, but still not be completely resistant to closure. Dilation with a single drop of the 10 % solution will likely be similar to that with two or more drops of the 2.5 % solution, only multiple drops of the 10 % solution are likely to produce a light-resistant pupil. Overall, recovery can still be expected in 24-36 h however.

(**vii**) effect of patient age on pharmacokinetics for phenylephrine eye drops; older patients tend to dilate better. Evidence suggests that the older a patient is the smaller their resting pupil might be, yet the smaller the resting pupil, the greater the relative dilation that can be achieved with phenylephrine eye drops. While the absolute dilated pupil size may not be any larger in older patients (compared with younger ones), the net dilation is greater.

(**viii**) effect of ocular pigmentation on pharmacokinetics of phenylephrine eye drops; pigment reduces efficacy. Evidence suggests that those individuals with darker pigmentation can show a slower response, and that the net dilation is 0.5 to 1 mm smaller than that for patients with lighter irides. As such, the solo use of eye drops containing phenylephrine 2.5 % in a patient with darkly pigmented eyes is of questionable value.

C. 6-hydroxyamphetamine eye drops. When used at the 1 % concentration, this is a special mydriatic with similar efficacy to eye drops containing phenylephrine 2.5 %. Commercial products are available in the USA, but could be prepared by a hospital pharmacy and used in the UK, in a hospital clinic.

D. OTHER DRUGS with mydriatic actions. Drugs such as cyclopentolate, homatropine, atropine, and hyoscine are marketed and should produce substantial mydriasis that is light resistant but are <u>not</u> normally indicated for use as diagnostic mydriatics due to an extended time base of action. They can be used however in therapeutic situations (see chapter 16) and as cycloplegics as an aid for refraction (Chapter 8).

E. COMBINATION MYDRIATICS, e.g. tropicamide plus phenylephrine. Over a 50 year period, numerous combinations of drugs in eye drops have either been tried, but no products are currently available in the UK. However, the desired effect can readily be achieved by instilling a single drop of <u>phenylephrine</u> 2.5 % and following it, 3 to 5 min later, with a single drop of <u>tropicamide</u> 1%. Pupil dilation follows a time course of action between that expected for phenylephrine or tropicamide alone. The pupil however now has two drugs acting upon it and a greater dilation (by 1 to 2 mm) can be achieved which resistant to light stimulation. Recovery from use of such a combination mydriatic is usually within 12 h, and often less.

SPECIAL CONSIDERATIONS IN THE USE OF MYDRIATICS

There are a number of factors that have been largely anecdotally documented to affect the efficacy of these drugs - either increasing or decreasing their efficacy, or making pupil dilation unpredictable either in terms of its onset, or its duration, and / or its magnitude or reversibility.

(**i**) the <u>diabetic patient</u>, especially type I; consider combination mydriatic because these pupils can be difficult to dilate. The diabetic pupil is likely to be slightly smaller in diabetics (esp. type II), and will be smaller still in patients with advanced stage diabetic retinopathy. The net result is that the pupil is resistant to dilation so two or more drops of tropicamide 1 % are needed to ensure adequate dilation. The diabetic pupil also may be more sensitive to phenylephrine, and so combinations should be used (providing there are no contraindications to the use of phenylephrine eye drops !).

(**ii**) the patient with <u>thyroid disorders</u>, especially hyperthyroidism (i.e. thyrotoxicosis in the extreme); tropicamide is the mydriatic of choice. The associated systemic conditions (e.g. high blood pressure and / or a predisposition to orthostatic hypotension) means that the combination eye drops should be used cautiously, especially because there may also be an increased systemic sensitivity to sympathomimetic drugs.

(**iii**) the <u>pregnant patient</u>; use tropicamide eye drops. Most pharmaceuticals carry a warning that safety in pregnancy has not been established. However, at those occasions when patient symptoms indicate the need to evaluate the peripheral fundus through a dilated pupil, the mydriatic should not be a sympathomimetic (e.g. phenylephrine) since systemic vasoconstrictor effects have been linked to transient fetal hypoxia.

(**iv**) the <u>postsurgical patient</u>; approach cautiously, do not expect routine dilation, but still consider dilating where appropriate. The general trauma of major systemic surgery may produce a general change in response to any autonomic drugs. However, providing there are no major post-operative complications, sensitivity to mydriatics can be expected to have normalized within 3 months. In cases of major ocular surgery (e.g. a corneal transplant for keratoconus), avoid dilating such patients in routine optometric practice for 2 to 3 months if any IOL has been implanted (unless requested to do so by a supervising ophthalmologist).

One special concern that has been voiced is that of the keratoconic patient wherein, following routine use of pre-operative mydriatics, the pupil dilates and stays dilated for weeks. While very rare, the dilated pupil is fixed and resistant to action of common miotics (e.g. pilocarpine 1 to 4 %), and so some recommend that such eyes should simply not be dilated in routine optometric practice. The mydriatic-induced condition is known as the Urrets-Zavalia syndrome.

(**v**) <u>patients on long-term ocular medical therapy</u>. With many types of therapies (with anti-infective drugs, anti-histamines, anti-inflammatory drugs etc.), there is no reason why the patient cannot be subjected to routine pupillary dilation. Other than allergies, it is most unlikely that any drug-drug interactions (**INT**) need to be considered. For the patient being medicated for ocular hypertension or glaucoma (see chapter 18), a few issues could be raised, but are minor compared to the need to perform a thorough eye examination. Visual fields assessments can be done following dilation, and some advocate that visual fields should be so assessed.

(**vi**) the <u>infected eye</u> (acute or subacute infection) and / or other diseases of the external eye. Infected and otherwise-diseased eyes should be dilated; use tropicamide. The patients require a little more attention, and instruments need special cleaning, but a mydriatic such as tropicamide can be used in most cases. If there are significant changes in corneal epithelium (e.g. associated with keratitis, keratoconjunctivitis, etc.), then the pharmacokinetics are likely to be faster and more extensive, so ensuring substantial mydriasis which can persist for a longer period. However, if the pupil is miotic because of concurrent inflammation, the enhanced penetration of the drug simply means that adequate dilation can be achieved.

NOTE. When dealing with the virus-infected eye, some have raised concerns for patients with a past history of <u>HSV keratitis</u>. It has been suggested that these of a sympathomimetic drug (e.g. phenylephrine, or epinephrine) may reactivate the virus; for routine diagnostic use, the use of phenylephrine is most unlikely to be a precipitating factor. For the infected eye, others have raised concerns that the use of mydriatic pharmaceuticals may delay wound healing of the corneal epithelium; for routine use of phenylephrine / tropicamide mydriatics, it is most unlikely that such effects could be of clinical consequence. The issue is relevant to a special use of phenylephrine 10 % eye drops, or cocaine 4 % eye drops, either of which may be used to "loosen" the corneal epithelium in cases with HSV keratitis.

(**vii**) other special disorders; approach cautiously, but still dilate - when there is a little more time available. Over the last 30 years, a number of groups of patients have been considered as being hypersensitive to the actions of mydriatics in the sense that the mydriatic (and cycloplegic) response was faster in onset, realized a greater than expected magnitude and lasted for a much longer period of time; none of these reports / claims have been fully documented. The patients include those with chronic migraine history, those with schizophrenia and perhaps other mental disorders, those with Alzheimer's, patients with Down's syndrome, patients with Marfan's syndrome, patients with MS (multiple sclerosis), patients with MH (malignant hyperthermia) and patients with epilepsy. Many of the "hypersensitivity" (supersensitivity) reports have actually involved the use of atropine eye drops rather than tropicamide or tropicamide-phenylephrine. Alternatively, these reports have arisen following the use of systemic medications (e.g. *i.v.* atropine, sympathomimetics in MH patients; barbiturates in epilepsy patients). In some cases, the issue specifically relates to local sensitivity to tropicamide eye drops only (e.g. Down's patients, or those with Alzheimer's), but a tropicamide eye drop test cannot be used to diagnose these conditions.

A similar scenario could easily develop for any patient who develops multiple allergies or general adverse reactions to drugs without there being any obvious reason for it. A GP is best advised / consulted prior to proceeding for the first time in such patients. One should be prepared to simply accept that a GP may simply decide that they do not want their patient dilated in the optometrists' office, e.g. patients with MH. An ophthalmologist or neurologist should then carry of the dilation.

(**viii**) the contact lens-wearing patient. Some have suggested that the pupil should dilate more since contact lens wear could compromise the structural integrity of the corneal epithelium. If there is punctate staining, enhanced drug permeation through the cornea could possibly occur.

(**ix**) use of topical ocular anaesthetics on the eye prior to use of a mydriatic will likely increase pupil dilation. Topical anaesthesia (e.g. proxymetacaine 0.5 % with fluorescein for applanation tonometry) will reduce the sensitivity of the ocular surface to the eye drop instillation, stinging symptoms should be markedly reduced and so reflex tearing will not wash the mydriatic out. The use of a single drop of any topical ocular anaesthetic some 5 min prior to the mydriatic drop(s) should produce a similar effect. Such a procedure may be useful in patients with epiphora, general reflex lacrimation (due to irritation etc.), or those apprehensive of the stinging effects of mydriatic eye drops. As a result, the mydriasis can be expected to be slightly larger (by 0.5 to 1 mm) or faster in onset. As with the regular use of topical ocular   . anaesthetics, it is important to always be aware of the possibility of adverse / hypersensitivity reactions (including to bisulphites).

OPHTHALMIC CYCLOPLEGIC DRUGS

Purpose of chapter. Select ocular drugs or pharmaceuticals produce substantial cycloplegia as well as mydriasis. Mydriatic drugs are widely used to facilitate examination of the inside of the eye. As a result of their mechanism of action, most mydriatics also produce an unwanted relaxation of the ciliary body, i.e. cycloplegia. It is largely this cycloplegic effect that needs to be remembered when considering patients' visual needs after mydriatic use. However, there are other situations where the cycloplegia is wanted as a desirable effect such that assessment of refractive error can be made, or the muscles are being relaxed to promote patient comfort. A full knowledge of the action of different cycloplegics is thus provided in this chapter to illustrate why only select drugs are used.

GENERAL CONSIDERATIONS FOR USE OF CYCLOPLEGICS

For the diagnostic use of cycloplegic drugs, the following patient aspects always need to be considered before decisions are made as to the use and / or management of a patient who has been "cyclopleged". All cycloplegic drugs cause substantial mydriasis so the use of cycloplegic drug is contraindicated in routine optometric practice in cases of known narrow angle glaucoma or in eyes that, on the basis of physical assessment, have a very narrow angle or the angle appears closed. While the chance of seeing such a restricted angle in a child is remote, the angle should still be evaluated; some special groups of patients who are routinely indicated for cycloplegic refraction may not have the same overall anatomical / ocular features as other children (e.g. Down's syndrome children). The use of cycloplegic eye drops is also contraindicated in cases of dislocation / subluxation of the crystalline lens, or predisposition to this (e.g. Marfan's syndrome, or patients with homocysteinura); such abnormal lens positioning should also be ruled out before (cycloplegic) refraction anyway. As with the use of mydriatics, the use of any cycloplegic should be approached with caution when the patient is on medications that may affect the pupil or the ciliary body; if the pupil is slightly dilated (via whatever mechanism), the prolonged action of most cycloplegics on the pupil may be even further lengthened. Similarly, if the ciliary body (accommodation) is affected, the interpretation and application of findings for the manifest refractive error versus those found under cycloplegia may be rather difficult, if not impossible. Patient rescheduling at a time when the medications have been discontinued or reduced, may be more appropriate for such patients. As with the use of mydriatics, and especially if refracting extremely young patients, consultation with the family physician may sometimes be appropriate if there is any reason to expect that the child may show an exaggerated reaction to the cycloplegic eye drops. For the therapeutic use of cycloplegics (Chapter 16), all of the above considerations are still important.

CYCLOPLEGIC DRUGS as DIAGNOSTIC AGENTS

Mechanisms. All clinically-used cycloplegic drugs are cholinergic blocking drugs. These drugs direct block the effects of acetylcholine at the muscle end-plates on ciliary muscles (as well as the iris sphincter muscle). These drugs are often referred to as anti-cholinergics or even as antimuscarinics because of a select blocking effect at muscarinic acetylcholine receptors.

A. Cyclopentolate [*sigh-cloe-pen-toh-late*] is the cycloplegic of choice for optometric practice and applicable to almost every situation and patient. Cyclopentolate can be used at either the 0.5 or 1% concentrations. A 2 % solution is marketed in the USA, but not in the UK.

(**i**) commercial products. Cyclopentolate is available as PoM **Minims**[R] **Cyclopentolate** as Eye-drops in the 0.5 % or 1 % concentration; the packets are stamped CYC 0.5 or CYC 1.0. Multi-use 5 mL bottles of cyclopentolate 0.5 % or 1 % are also available (PoM **Mydrilate**[R] Eye Drops).

NOTE. Some hospitals may use a specially-prepared ophthalmic spray for administration of cyclopentolate to children. The children are usually asked to lightly close their eyes and the small dispenser is used to spray a known quantity of solution onto the eyelid margins; the child is asked to open their eyes and the 'drops' go in. The dispenser is not currently commercially available for general use.

(**ii**) ingredients. The eye drops contain cyclopentolate 0.5 or 1 %. The nature of the aqueous vehicle is such that the eye drops can sting markedly on instillation. The **Minims**[R] products are preservative-free, while the preservative in multi-use bottles is benzalkonium chloride. Cyclopentolate eye drops should be stored in a cool place, but refrigeration is not generally recommended. On degradation, the solutions may turn very pale brown or a straw color, but is not known to form precipitates. The limited external signs of deterioration thus means that the expiration date is especially important.

(**iii**) indicated for use whenever there are variable or inconsistent refraction results that are attributed either to inadequate control of accommodation, uncertainty in the extent of patient cooperation with the refraction, or in conditions where the apparent refractive error condition is linked to periodic or persistent strabismus (especially esotropia's).

(**iv**) contraindications (**C/I**) specific for cyclopentolate is known sensitivity to the drug, or any of its ingredients.

(**v**) special precautions (**S/P**) in any patient with any form or history of central neurological disorders, to include disorders of motor coordination associated with developing disease or after severe trauma. The use of cyclopentolate-containing eye drops can very occasionally precipitate an "immediate" (i.e. within 5-10 min of eye drop instillation) CNS-based reaction. As a result, CNS-linked symptoms and behavioural changes (including disorientation perceptual changes, hallucinations, rapid speech changes, uncontrolled limb movements or even collapse) can occur. The responses can be expected to be self-limiting without any long-lasting effects. The patient should be monitored, first aid administered; that the reaction occurred should be noted in the patients' records !.

The reaction /behaviour may be the result of an unusually large systemic absorption of the cyclopentolate that occurs via the conjunctival mucous membranes, and so punctal occlusion etc., is not a viable means for "preventing" the problem. These behavioural responses to cycloplegic eye drops have been reported for other cholinergic blockers (including hyoscine, atropine and homatropine) but have been more commonly reported with cyclopentolate. The individual patient reaction is not predictable and there do not appear to be any particular predisposing factors. The reaction(s) can occur with any dose of cyclopentolate, but it is generally considered that the risk is highest if the 2 % solution is used; this 2 % product is thus not recommended for use in children. Many recommend that cyclopentolate should not be for domiciliary use in infants and children.

(vi) pharmacokinetics for cyclopentolate eye drops. A minimum dose equivalent to that found in a single drop of the 1 % solution (or 2 drops of the 0.5 % solution) should be used. This may be achieved with the single drop or with two drops of 0.5% solution, separated by an interval of 5 to 10 minutes. For refraction of a child (i.e. aged 5 to 8 yrs), it is essential that enough drug is used to ensure adequate relaxation of the ciliary body. With the dose specified, the amplitude of accommodation can be expected to be reduced, in most patients, to < 2.0 D within 30 minutes (at which time cycloplegic refraction can be performed). The recovery from cycloplegia is relatively slow, with limited reading ability returning in 4 to 8 hrs but with full recovery taking 12 to 24 h. It should be noted that the pupil usually remains dilated for a further 12 to 24 hrs after the full recovery from cycloplegia, and appropriate patient /parent counselling is important.

(vii) pharmacokinetics and patient age for cyclopentolate. While there is no reported age-dependent effect per se, a simple rule can be adopted in that the larger and more dynamic the initial amplitude of accommodation, the more resistant the accommodation mechanism will be to the action of the cycloplegic drug. For example, in younger children of just 3 to 5 yrs, residual amplitudes of 3 to 4 D may exist even 30 minutes after cyclopentolate 1 % use, and so the dosage may need to be increased to 2 gtt 1 % or 3 gtt 0.5 % etc. For children under 3 yrs, the dose can probably be the same as for 3 to 5 year-olds. There is good evidence to suggest that the instilled doses do NOT need to be any higher, providing that child / infant does not cry the drug out !. In pre-teens and early teens, the residual amplitude after use of cyclopentolate 1% is usually less than 2 D. For patients over 15 years, the dose of a single drop of cyclopentolate 1 % should almost always be adequate. For patients over 30 years of age, a single drop of the 0.5 % solution should be adequate.

(**viii**) effect of <u>ocular pigmentation</u> on pharmacokinetics of cyclopentolate. There is substantial clinical evidence to show that the darker the ocular pigmentation of a patient, then the slower the onset and the less pronounced the net cycloplegic effects are after the instillation of cyclopentolate. In addition, the darker the pigmentation, the slower the recovery from cycloplegia. Appropriate dosage adjustment is thus necessary, e.g. a minimum dose of 2 *gtt* cyclopentolate 1 % in children (5 to 8 years of age) with very dark irides. The slow recovery is attributed to a slow release of the drug from ocular pigment and this slow recovery may be particularly frustrating for a child anxious to get out and play again!.

Cyclopentolate is clearly the drug of choice for cycloplegic refraction. There are some alternatives available however and that can be considered for some patients in optometric practices.

B. Homatropine eye drops can be considered as an alternative cycloplegic for children where there is known or suspected sensitivity to cyclopentolate, or where home-instillation of the cycloplegic is considered preferable to instilling eye drops in the office just prior to a refraction. The latter situation might include cases where the irritation associated with cyclopentolate instillation is too traumatic to allow continuance of an examination. Homatropine eye drops, while they may produce temporary but rather marked vasodilatation of the conjunctiva, may not sting as much as cyclopentolate eye drops.

(**i**) <u>commercial products</u>. PoM **Minims**^{R} **Homatropine Hydrobromide** Eye-drops in single-use containers; the package is stamped HOM 2.0. Multi-use 10 mL bottles (PoM **Homatropine** Eye-drops, generic) are also available at both the 1 % and 2 % concentration.

(**ii**) <u>ingredients</u> include homatropine 1 or 2 %. The **Minims**^{R} product is preservative-free while multi-use products will be preserved with benzalkonium chloride or benzethonium chloride. The products are not expected to show obvious signs of deterioration when degraded etc., so expiration date is important. Store at room temperature; do not refrigerate.

(**iii**) <u>contraindications</u> (**C/I**) for the use of homatropine include known hypersensitivity to the drug or any of the ingredients of the eye drops. As with cyclopentolate, special precautions (**S/P**) in the use of homatropine eye drops should include patients who are on medications that produce mydriasis. If these same medications exert even mild cycloplegic effects, as with cyclopentolate use, the diagnostic use of homatropine is unlikely to be productive. The use of homatropine eye drops has also been reported to be associated with CNS effects, but less commonly than with cyclopentolate. If the homatropine has been prescribed for domiciliary use (e.g. by providing a parent with, several **Minims**^{R} products or the multi-use bottle) then it is a good idea to check that the appropriate dosing was administered before the refraction; any un-used products should also be returned at the time of the refraction.

(**iv**) pharmacokinetics of homatropine eye drops. The action of homatropine on the ciliary body is relatively slow when compared to cyclopentolate, especially in children or teenagers. This slowness in onset is however unlikely to be of any clinical consequence since multiple drops of homatropine should be used. If the 2 % concentration is used, at least three and perhaps up to five drops should be instilled with an interval of 10 to 15 minutes between the drops. When the 1 % concentration is used, five drops administered over 12 hrs would be the indicated regimen and dose. The residual accommodation, providing adequate doses are used, can be expected to be < 2.0 D even in children. Recovery, such that reasonable near point vision is restored (but not necessarily adequate for reading) is slow, e.g. 24 to 48 h for 3 *gtt* of homatropine 2 %. The pupil dilation can be expected to out-last the cycloplegic effects by 2 to 3 days in many children.

(**iv**) effects of patient age on pharmacokinetics of homatropine eye drops. Treat as for cyclopentolate.

(**v**) effects of ocular pigmentation on pharmacokinetics of homatropine eye drops. Treat as for cyclopentolate. Some have suggested that multiple drops, of homatropine are especially useful in with very densely pigmented eyes, e.g. for Afro-Carribean individuals.

C. Atropine. Some individuals still consider atropine to be the cycloplegic of choice in children under 4 years of age, or for those with substantial accommodative esotropia. For the latter case, this may be true because prolonged and substantial cycloplegia may be what is needed to uncover the source of the esotropia. However, numerous reports have indicated that satisfactory refraction can be achieved on patients all the way down to the age of 4 months following the use of cyclopentolate 0.5 or 1 %. The continued diagnostic use of atropine thus seems unnecessary.

(i) Commercial products. PoM **Minims**[R] **Atropine Sulphate** 1 % Eye-drops in single use containers; the packages are stamped ATRO 1.0. Multi-use 5 mL bottles of atropine 1 % are available as PoM **Isopto Atropine**[R]); multi-use 10 mL bottles of atropine 0.5 % or 1 % are available as generics (PoM **Atropine**[R], or PoM **Atropine Sulphate**[R], generic). A 3 g tube of atropine ointment 1 % (PoM **Atropine**[R], generic) is also available.

(ii) ingredients. The Minims[R] product contains atropine 1 % and is non-preserved. Eye drops in multi-use bottles contain atropine 0.5 or 1 % and are preserved with benzalkonium chloride; the ointment is also preserved with benzalkonium chloride.

(iii) <u>contraindications</u> (**C/I**) for the use of atropine eye drops or eye ointments include known hypersensitivity to the drug or any of the ingredients of the pharmaceutical. Special precautions (**S/P**) for use of ophthalmic atropine should be consideration of concurrent use of any medications with atropine-like drugs; for children, this is likely to include stomach medications and anti-diarrhoeal agents, e.g. oral hyoscine ([*high-oh-seen*], P **Buscopan**[R], see below); oral diphenoxylate ([*dye-fen-ox'i-late*], PoM **Lomotil**[R]). As with cyclopentolate, it is not possible to stop systemic absorption of atropine. (**ADR**) The important signs and symptoms to look out with domiciliary atropine use are those associated with a mild systemic "overdose" wherein all the predictable parasympatholytic effects can develop, and sometimes acutely, e.g. dry mouth (thirsty), reduction in sweating (feels hot and may look flushed), increased pulse (agitated, excited and also flushed) and reduction in GI tract motility (constipated); urinary retention can occur as well. These effects will be self-limiting in that they will subside as the drug is eliminated from the body. Smaller children should be considered for lower doses, i.e. use the 0.5 % drops instead of the 1 %. Since urinary retention can occur, atropine eye drops should be used cautiously in children medicated with cholinergic blocking drugs for incontinence (e.g. oral oxybutynin [*ox-ee-byoo'ti-nin*], PoM **Cystrin**[R]).

(iv) <u>pharmacokinetics</u> for atropine eye drops. When used as a diagnostic agent, atropine is meant to be used repeatedly, and at home. Commonly recommended doses are one or two drops (depending on how well the first drop went in) and to repeat this morning and evening for 2 days prior to examination and then a last set of drops is instilled on the morning of the eye examination. In resistant children or those prone to crying, some recommend use of the ointment on the same schedule. With this type of dosing, the accommodation should be reduced to 2 D by the end of the first day but the reason for use of atropine is so that the accommodation stays relaxed to uncover the esotropia. Recovery can be expected to take a full week or more because of the repeated application of the eye drops or ointment (although even a single drop of atropine 1 % can reduce accommodation for several days in older individuals).

(**v**) effects of <u>age</u> and <u>ocular pigmentation</u> on pharmacokinetics of atropine eyedrops or ointments. Treat as for cyclopentolate.

Since the atropine is often for domiciliary use, it is a good idea to get the parent to return any unused eye drops or ointment. This also provides an opportunity to check that the right dose was used and to make a note of any adverse reactions that were encountered.

D. Hyoscine [*high-oh-seen*]. This is another direct acting-cholinergic blocker that was available in a 10 mL multi-use bottle as PoM **Hyoscine** (generic) 0.25 % eye-drops; such eye drops could still be prepared by a · major hospital pharmacy (and probably be preserved with benzalkonium chloride). It could be considered for patients that show allergic reactions to other cycloplegics (e.g. cyclopentolate) but can produce the same type of systemic parasympatholytic effects. The pharmacokinetics are similar to the use of atropine 1 % eye drops.

E. Tropicamide eye drops are indicated for cycloplegic refraction only in "older" patients with lesser amplitudes of accommodation (< 8 D).

(i) commercial products. PoM **Minims**^R **Tropicamide** Eye Drops containing tropicamide 1 %; the packs are marked TRO 1.0.

(ii) ingredients. Tropicamide 1 % and the **Minims**^R are preservative free. The aqueous vehicle is such that the eye drops can sting somewhat on instillation. The product should not be refrigerated.

(iii) indications for use as a cycloplegic. Infrequent, but can be (should be?) considered for a patient older than 25 yrs (where a dosage equivalent to 1 *gtt* of the 1 % solution can almost certainly be expected to produce the necessary relaxation of accommodation). If one is to use tropicamide as a cycloplegic, then one really should not be doing so when the patients amplitude is such that multiple drops are needed (because cyclopentolate. would likely be more effective). Despite this, some of those concerned over toxicity reactions to cyclopentolate advocate the routine use of 3 *gtt* tropicamide 1 % for paediatric cycloplegia.

(iv) contraindications (**C/I**) specific for the use of tropicamide are known sensitivity to the tropicamide or any other ingredients.

(v) special precautions (**S/P**) for use of tropicamide in patients on medications that produce mydriasis, especially in those approaching presbyopia (37 to 40 yrs) where an exaggerated or sustained pupil dilation could cause substantial visual problems for daily activities.

(vi) pharmacokinetics for tropicamide eye drops as a cycloplegic. In patients older than 25 yrs, a single drop of tropicamide 1 % can be expected to reduce the amplitude of accommodation to less than 2 D in 15 to 20 minutes. The maximal effect is however relatively brief in many patients (i.e. only 10 to 20 minutes for maximum cycloplegia), so careful timing of the refractions is important. Recovery is rapid and reasonable reading ability can be expected in 1 to 2 hrs.

(vii) effect of patient age on pharmacokinetics of tropicamide eye drops. Tropicamide, as a cycloplegic, is best only used in patients with only moderate amplitudes (e.g.< 8 D). Such amplitudes are most frequently found in patients aged 25 to 40 yrs of age. The older the patient, the more complete the action of tropicamide (as a cycloplegic) can be expected to be.

(**viii**) effect of <u>ocular pigmentation</u> on pharmacokinetics of tropicamide eye drops. The cycloplegic action of tropicamide is clearly pigment-dependent. The greater the level of pigmentation, the lesser the cycloplegia that can be expected. With increasing pigment, the speed of onset of adequate cycloplegia and the depth of cycloplegia can be expected to be less. With very darkly pigmented eyes, residual amplitudes of much greater than 2 D can be expected (even with multiple drops of tropicamide 1 %); use cyclopentolate 1 %for such eyes.

NOTE on the cycloplegic effects of sympthomimetics such as phenylephrine. For most older individuals (young adults), evidence from clinical studies suggests that the neural control of their accommodation is predominantly under parasympathetic control. This means that, functionally, all of their accommodative functions can be 'blocked' with the appropriate of a cholinergic blocking drug. It should be noted however that some of the neural control for accommodation is sympathetic and thus the measured near-point amplitude of accommodation can be reduced with the instillation of phenylephrine eye drops. Combination cycloplegics containing phenylephrine and a hyoscine-like drug are marketed in the USA, specifically for paediatric cycloplegic refractions.

THERAPEUTIC USES OF MYDRIATICS AND CYCLOPLEGICS

When certain diseases of the eye develop, there are special uses of cycloplegic-mydriatic drugs, especially for atropine. These uses are para-therapeutic and a substantial extension of the use of these drugs for diagnostic purposes. However, the use of such cycloplegic-mydriatic / mydriatic-cycloplegic drugs is part of a normal standard of care for eyes with inflammation, or at risk for developing inflammation. The reaction of the eye to cycloplegics can be expected to be rather different in the inflamed eye (see chapter 16), although the same pharmacodynamic principles apply. Atropine and homatropine are the standard cycloplegics for therapeutic use, although - for older patients with uveitis (or similar) - cyclopentolate can still be used because of its substantial cycloplegic effect, but the repeated use of cyclopentolate is to be avoided in infants and young children.

MIOTICS

Purpose of chapter. Miotics are a specific group of drugs that have a number of clinical uses because of their ability to close down the pupil. Their main use is in the long-term management of ocular hypertension in some types of open-angle glaucoma, along with other drugs that can be used to lower IOP. They are also used as part of the management of angle-closure glaucoma. In this chapter, the various miotic drugs will be discussed, and the reasons for their selection and clinical use outlined.

As with all ocular pharmaceutical agents, no miotic should be used when there is known hypersensitivity to the miotic or any ingredients of the pharmaceutical. Notwithstanding, even with single dose applications to the eye, the use of miotics is often perceived to carry much higher risks than the use of other diagnostic drugs. Similarly, the chronic use of miotics has a higher incidence of precipitating ocular ADR's (that are severe enough to warrant discontinuation of the use of the eyedrops) than most other ophthalmic drugs.

MECHANISMS OF MIOTIC ACTION

From a clinical perspective, there are three ways in which a miotic can close the pupil. Direct-acting (muscarinic) cholinergics close the pupil by contracting the iris sphincter muscle; indirect-acting cholinergics produce the same effect. Direct-acting *alpha*-adrenergic blocking drugs produce miosis as a result of relaxing the iris dilator muscle by blocking the normal action of norepinephrine that would contract the dilator muscle; with the dilator muscle relaxed, the pupil then closes under the action of the normal light reflex of the sphincter muscle. Alternatively, pharmacodynamic data suggests that activation of inhibitory $alpha_2$ receptors will also block the action of norepinephrine on the dilator and so produce miosis. The adrenergic/ adrenergic blocking drugs are all low potency, low efficacy miotics compared to the cholinergic miotics. Indirect-acting cholinergic drugs are anti-cholinesterases, increase acetylcholine levels around the iris sphincter muscle, to produce a stronger and more prolonged contraction than that observed after use of the direct-acting cholinergic drugs.

PRODUCTS CONTAINING MIOTICS

(a) pilocarpine - a direct-acting cholinergic which has been used for over 100 years, and the miotic most likely used by an optometrist. It is routinely available as eye drops in a number of concentrations, e.g. 0.5 to 4 %. The range of concentrations allow for selection of just the right strength of this miotic for the particular clinical situation. Currently available pharmaceuticals include PoM **Minims**R **Pilocarpine Nitrate** Eye-drops (1, 2 and 4 %) in unit-dose containers. A range of other pilocarpine products are also available (see chapter 18).

(**b**) carbachol [*kar-ba'-koll*] - a direct-acting cholinergic drug, used to lower IOP. It is one alternative to pilocarpine, if local irritation develops with sustained use of pilocarpine eye drops. Carbachol eye drops are currently only available at the 3 % concentration (i.e. PoM **Isopto Carbachol**[R] in a 10 mL multi-use bottle).

(**c**) apraclonidine [*a-pra-cloe-ni-deen*] - an *alpha*$_2$ adrenergic drug. Available in preservative-free unit-dose preparations (PoM **Iopidine**[R], for use by ophthalmologists pre- and post-operatively), and in 5 ml multi-use bottles (as a pre-operative alternative to pilocarpine; see chapter 18).

(**d**) echothiophate [*ekko-thye-o'-fate*] - an indirect-acting cholinergic, which is a largely-irreversible (i.e. very long lasting) inhibitor of acetylcholinesterase. It had a high potential for producing systemic parasympathetic ADR's following conjunctival absorption. It was once generally available as PoM **Phospholine Iodide**[R] Eye-drops (0.06, 0.125 and 0.25%). These are no longer generally marketed in the UK but are available on a named-patient basis through a hospital. It is thus reserved for very selective use only when other miotics fail to produce the desired clinical response.

(**e**) demecarium [*dem-ec-air-ee-um*] - an indirect-acting cholinergic, also with largely-irreversible actions and thus a high potential for parasympathetic ADR's. It was marketed as PoM **Tosmilen**[R] Eye-drops at the 0.125 and 0.5 % concentrations but now, like echothiophate, is only available on a named-patient basis for use under strict supervision when other miotics fail to produce the desired effects.

(**f**) physostigmine [*fye-soh-stig-meen*] - an indirect-acting cholinergic. Was usually used at the 0.25 % concentration, as eye drops but no products are currently listed as it is rarely used. Generics (e.g. PoM **Physostigmine**, in a 10 mL multi-use bottle) were listed. It could be used by optometrists.

(**g**) DFP (= diisopropylfluorophosphate, isoflurophate, difluorophate, dyflos) - an indirect-acting and irreversible acetylcholinesterase inhibitor. It had a similar use to and similar limitations to use as echothiophate but is no longer used in the UK.

(**h**) thymoxamine [*thye-mox-ah-meen*] - a direct-acting *alpha*-adrenergic blocking drug. This drug was available for many years (as PoM **Minims**[R] **Thymoxamine** Eye-drops 0.5 %) but is no longer available. Thymoxamine was generally indicated for use after a pupil has been dilated with phenylephrine 10 %, and it could be used by optometrists.

(**i**) dapiprazole [*da-pip-ra'-zole*]- a direct-acting *alpha-* adrenergic blocking drug. Not marketed in UK, but eye drops containing dapiprazole 0.5 % are marketed in Europe (e.g. GLAMIDOLO[R] in Italy) and the USA (e.g. REV-EYES[R]). Where available, dapiprazole is specifically indicated for use after a pupil has been dilated with tropicamide or phenylephrine / tropicamide combinations (see later).

PREPARATION and CARE OF MIOTICS

A number of miotics require special handling. A good rule for miotics therefore is to store them all in a cool, dark and dry place when not in use. Even if supplied in unit dose containers or standard multi-use white plastic bottles (e.g. pilocarpine), these eye drops containing miotics should not be exposed to continuous light. Echothiophate eye drops are only available in special amber bottles, as a powder to be reconstituted with a sterile solution (provided with the bottles) to give concentrations of 0.06, 0.125 and 0.25%. The reconstituted product had to be used within 3 weeks if stored at room temperature, or within 3 months if refrigerated. As currently marketed in Europe, dapiprazole is provided as a powder, in a special bottle, that needs to be reconstituted prior to use with a special solution (that is supplied with the bottle). The resultant solution should be used within 21 days, and kept refrigerated at all times.

PHARMACOKINETICS and GENERAL EFFECTS OF MIOTICS

(i) the efficacy of all miotics is markedly dependent upon the level of ocular pigmentation; the darker or more intense the pigmentation, the lesser the efficacy of the miotics. The most frequent reason presented for this effect is that the ocular pigment binds the miotic drug and thus reduces the quantity of drug available for binding to the receptors (including enzymes) on the iris, ciliary body or ciliary epithelium.

(ii) pharmacokinetics. The onset of miosis will be very dependent upon the concentration of the miotic used (e.g. pilocarpine) with lower concentrations requiring 30 min for a miosis (to close the pupil to c. 2 mm) to occur while high concentrations may produce the same full miosis in 15 min. Apraclonidine, dapiprazole and thymoxamine are "weaker" miotics and do not produce much miosis, while physostigmine, echothiophate, demecarium and DFP act as if higher concentrations (>4 %) of pilocarpine were being used.

(iii) pupillary light responses are usually slowed and are essentially absent after the appropriate degree of miosis has been elicited for the concentration used. The miotic drug has the dominant effect on the pupil and 'fixes' it at a certain diameter which is unlikely to change when the light levels are increased or decreased.

(iv) ciliary body effects. The cholinergic miotics (direct or indirect-acting) also increase the tone of the ciliary body by causing part of the ciliary muscle to contract. As a result a pseudomyopia or simply a relative pseudomyopic shift can occur in 'younger' individuals. The term pseudomyopia is used because the shift will reverse when the drug effects wear off. Changes of several dioptres are easily realised in younger eyes, but there is little effect in older eyes. The sustained contraction can cause eye dtrain and a headache. The effects should be manifest in 30 minutes and take 1 to 4 h to wear off if single dosing is used. For repeated dosing, an adaptation occurs over a few days so lesser effects occur. The adrenergic blocking miotics are unlikely to produce substantial effects on the ciliary body but are capable of affecting it. From a theoretical perspective, some individuals have stated that the ciliary body should not be affected by $alpha_1$-blockers but there is not good clinical data to support this concept.

(**v**) the rate of aqueous production will probably be decreased by direct-acting cholinergic miotics, and by apraclonidine. For the cholinergic miotics, this effect is additive to them generally increasing outflow facility by opening up the trabecular meshwork (see below). Apraclonidine appears to have a specific effect on reducing aqueous production, but it is uncertain whether the alpha-adrenergic blocking drugs reduce aqueous secretion.

(**vi**) the depth of the anterior chamber should decrease after the use of cholinergic miotics, while adrenergic drugs are unlikely to produce a clinically-measurable effect on anterior chamber depth.

(**vii**) IOP should fall after the use of any miotic. The effect is, attributed to the miosis which, via the scleral spur, should mechanically open up the outflow facility. If little miosis develops with the use of a miotic, little ocular hypotensive effect can be expected.

(**viii**) All miotics, directly or indirectly, cause vasodilatation. This effect is usually accompanied by a marked "smarting" response and the *alpha*-adrenergic blocking drugs are renowned for this unwanted effect. The resulting vasodilatation can produce a marked conjunctival hyperaemia that persists for several hours after the eye drops were instilled. With repeated use, miotics can produce marked congestion of the conjunctival vasculature that is both uncomfortable and cosmetically unappealing.

CONTRAINDICATIONS (**C/I**)
FOR THE USE OF MIOTICS in ROUTINE OPTOMETRIC PRACTICE

These can essentially be summarised by the term "when miosis is undesirable" as a result of the risk of adverse reactions developing, i.e.

(**i**) patients with known allergy to the miotic solution.

(**ii**) patients who have had an iridectomy, iridotomy or related procedure in the last year; the miotic could alter the patency of such surgery.

(**iii**) patients with iris-supported intra-ocular lenses; the use of the miotic may displace the lens or tear the iris tissue.

(**iv**) patients with intra-ocular inflammation where there is marked iris involvement (iritis); these conditions may be associated with scleritis, anterior or posterior uveitis, general iris neovascularisation (including rubeosis). The miotic may precipitate pupil block (iris *bombe*) and / or cause unacceptably large release of pigment from the iris.

(**v**) patients with a marked history of, or presenting with, posterior synechiae. These patients may be given or prescribed miotics by an ophthalmologist, but this use is best done in a clinic where there is surgical support available (in case iris / pupil block occurs).

(**vi**) patients with known <u>exfoliative disorders of the crystalline lens</u>. Always check the lens margins after dilating an older patient or where there is marked pigmentary loss from the iris (transillumination). The use of a miotic in such patients may produce pupil block. This limitation may not apply to the adrenergic drugs.

(**vii**) <u>Lens subluxation</u>. Miotics should be used with caution or avoided when there are any disorders of the lens that could alter the position of the lens in the eye. These include cases of lens subluxation and patients with a very shallow anterior chamber. In these types of cases, pupil block may result from use of a miotic. This limitation may not apply to the adrenergic drugs.

(**viii**) patients with history of or presenting signs and symptoms of <u>retinal detachment</u> or indications of retinal traction. While this limitation to use really only applies to the use of indirect-acting cholinergics, the risk of a miotic precipitating retinal traction is obviously one that can be avoided if miotics are not used. This limitation may not apply to the adrenergic drugs.

CLINICAL USES OF MIOTICS

(**i**) TO REVERSE A MYDRIATIC PUPIL following use of mydriatics (or mydriatic - cycloplegics). A tropicamide, or phenylephrine- tropicamide-dilated pupil can be very readily "closed" with pilocarpine 1 % or 2 % (1 or 2 drops, separated by a 5 min interval). If available, physostigmine 0.25 % (1 or 2 drops, separated by a 5 min interval), could be used. When thymoxamine was used, the standard dosing was 1 to 3 drops. For dapiprazole 0.5 % eye-drops, the standard dosing is 4 drops, separated by a few minutes each. Other miotics produce similar effects but are generally not indicated for this use.

Use-related issues. Overall, this use of a miotic was commonplace in the days when short-acting mydriatics (e.g. tropicamide) were not available. The procedure is really not necessary after phenylephrine 2.5 % (although it was once widely done following phenylephrine 10 % use) or 6-hydroxy - amphetamine 1 % eye drops. When a miotic is used to close down a dilated pupil, the pupil should return to nearly its pre-mydriatic size in about 1 hour. The use of a miotic to close a pupil is an approved procedure for optometrists in the UK, but this approval should be recognised as being logically restricted to the use of eye drops, e.g. those containing pilocarpine.

Some clinicians have suggested that a dilated pupil *per se* may be especially bothersome to hyperopes due to the associated mild cycloplegia and so these patients should be closed after use of a mydriatic. This theoretically would allow a patient to leave the eye examination with better vision than if they left partially or fully dilated. If the miotic was used on a younger patient, both cholinergic miotics and adrenergic-blocking miotics have been also shown to hasten the recovery of accommodation after use of tropicamide or tropicamide-phenylephrine. It must be noted however that the "overuse" of a miotic after the routine (and uneventful) use of mydriatics can produce a pupil size that is smaller than before the patient was dilated; a slightly miotic pupil, in itself, can cause vision problems.

Safety issues. A number of issues have been discussed concerning this procedure. In using a miotic (e.g. pilocarpine) to close a pupil, it should be noted that the relative speed of pupil closure towards the crystalline lens (if present) coupled with forward movement of the crystalline lens (especially if the patient is not presbyopic) is considered to place the eye into a potential position for a pupil block (iris *bombe*, iris seclusion); the mid-dilated position is considered to be that at which the greatest risk is present. Hyperopes and / or those with a shallow anterior chamber (perhaps associated with a plateau iris) are considered to be more at risk. The concern has been mainly voiced over the use of pilocarpine (or other cholinergic miotics).The use of the *alpha*-adrenergic blocking drugs has been considered to have substantially less potential to precipitate a pupil block, and these were once strongly promoted as "safe miotics".

 The risks for a pupil block are considered much less for a pupil dilated with stronger cholinergic blocking drugs (e.g. homatropine, cyclopentolate, hyoscine or atropine) simply because the miotic has to counter (reverse) the strong cholinergic blocking drug action first, before being able to produce miosis. With pronounced cycloplegic actions of homatropine etc., the cycloplegic action has to be reversed first, before any lens movement is likely to occur. A pupil block could however develop without lens movement if there is a substantially thickened lens, exfoliation or posterior synechiae. All of these however contrast to a situation where phenylephrine-tropicamide (or tropicamide alone) has been used as the mydriatic and for which the resistance to miosis is minimal and rapid pupil closure can occur.

(ii) TO MANAGE ANGLE CLOSURE following use of a mydriatic (with ensuing elevation in IOP) or an "off-the-street" angle closure patient (where the angle closure could have been precipitated by systemic medications). The use of a miotic has been considered to be an essential part of the management of angle closure for over 50 years, regardless of the aetiology of the angle closure. The use of a miotic to manage angle closure should be addressed from the perspective of the etiology of the angle closure, i.e. iatrogenic or natural (spontaneous). Some have argued that the use of a miotic in such cases could exacerbate the condition by worsening a pupil block situation; others clearly disagree !. Periodically, other ideas have been voiced. However, in common with those general concerns that miotics should not be used, these ideas have not been supported by substantial clinical observations (i.e. case histories or unambiguous prospective studies). In addition, it can be noted that while other types of pharmacological management of angle closure may well have some positive effects (see later), the key question to be addressed is whether these other drugs can be used on the average patient who experiences angle closure. The answer is a definite yes!.

(a) <u>angle closure precipitated by a mydriatic-cycloplegic</u>. In reality, pilocarpine is the most likely miotic to be used, unless the pupil fails to respond. In using a miotic to manage an iatrogenic angle closure, it is most important that the <u>dose</u> of the miotic chosen should be commensurate with the <u>severity</u> of the condition. Therefore, for pilocarpine eye drops, the concentration chosen must be commensurate with the "strength" of the mydriatic that precipitated the condition. For example, at least 2 % and perhaps 4 % pilocarpine would be needed to effectively reverse a cyclopentolate-dilated pupil. Lower concentrations (1 or 2 %) might be used following dilation with tropicamide, or following dilation with phenylephrine-tropicamide. In each case, the higher concentration would be used in those with darkly pigmented eyes. Conversely, some clinicians have expressed such great concern about the risk of precipitating pupil block that they advocate the use of pilocarpine 0.5 % (e.g. PoM **Isopto Carpine**[R], in a 10 mL multi-use bottle); detailed case histories showing the efficacy of such a use do not appear to have been published however.

The time-honoured <u>dosing schedule</u> was to instill a drop of miotic q 15 min until the angle has opened. This should result in the IOP starting to decrease (verified by tonometry if possible) and the angle being reopened (verified by pen-light or slit lamp, but perhaps being more difficult to assess in such situations). For some patients, 1 or 2 drops are sufficient to 'break the attack'; in other patients, 4 or 6 drops might be required. If a pupil fails to respond to repeated instillation of pilocarpine eye drops, physostigmine eye drops should produce the same effect. In a hospital setting, even stronger miotics such as echothiophate would likely be tried in unresponsive cases.

(b) <u>spontaneous angle closure</u>. These can occur completely spontaneously (and be probably associated with a history of intermittent closure) or be associated with the use of systemic medications (see chapter 10). In such cases, while signs and symptoms may be just as substantial as following an iatrogenic angle closure, the attack is usually far easier to break. The miotic dose used should still be commensurate with the degree of ocular pigmentation, and the miotic should be presented until the attack is broken. Usually the more dilute concentrations (e.g. 1 or 2 %) of pilocarpine will suffice and only 1 or 2 drops are likely to be needed.

SUPPLEMENTARY MEDICATIONS for ANGLE CLOSURE

The use of a miotic will usually open the angle (and must do so) but may not lower the intra-ocular pressure fast enough; sustained elevation in IOP (i.e. above 50 mm Hg) carries the risk of producing long-term damage to the retina and nerve head, as well as permanently damaging the corneal endothelium. Therefore, the adjunct use of a variety of other ocular hypotensive agents is generally recommended, unless the patient cannot tolerate them. Some of these measures have been proposed, by some, to be effective as the sole measure for managing angle-closure glaucoma but there is little published evidence to support these proposals. Therefore, while some of these "supplementary" (adjunct) measures may be effective monotherapy on a case-by-case basis, they should not be assumed to be general primary measures to manage angle closure glaucoma.

(**i**) oral glycerin. This is an emergency adjunct medication when access to other adjunct medications / treatments is limited or difficult. It is meant for a single use only as part of a management that includes prompt referral to a physician. It is not recommended for use in diabetics (as its use could precipitate severe hyperglycaemia). The patient should be instructed to drink / sip 100 to 200 mL of the liquid reasonably rapidly (i.e. over 5 min). This procedure is generally not recommended for diabetic patients. The glycerin is an extremely sweet, syrupy liquid that is a Pharmacy Medicine, e.g. as a 50, 100, 250 or 500 mL bottle labelled as glycerin(e) or glycerol. It should be stored in a refrigerator at all times once opened. The viscous liquid should be mixed 1:1 with fruit juice (over ice if that is preferred) and the measure of 100 to 200 mL should be sufficient. It should be noted that the patient may find the drink produces nausea, and has been known to cause vomiting. The IOP should start to fall within 15 to 30 min after ingestion of the syrupy solution and be approaching normal values within an hour. Such uses of oral glycerol can be effective on IOP's as high as 60 mm Hg. Since glycerol is also an osmotic diuretic, a patient may need to urinate just about at that time when you wish to start re-taking IOP's, i.e. 30 min later.

(**ii**) oral acetazolamide [*ah-seet-ah-zoll-a-mide*] This is generally considered to be the best adjunct medication for angle closure glaucoma, providing there are no contraindications to its use. The commercial product is PoM **Diamox**^R supplied as tablets containing 250 mg acetazolamide; generic 250 mg tablets (PoM **Acetazolamide**) are also generally available. The most widely accepted dose is 500 mg (i.e. 2 x 250 mg taken with a small quantity of water); only one such dose is usually required.

Acetazolamide is a diuretic and also acts as a specific inhibitor of aqueous secretion because it inhibits the enzyme carbonic anhydrase that is present in the ciliary epithelium. The IOP should start to fall within 30 min, and its administration will likely prompt urination within 15 to 30 min. A single dose can be effective on IOP's as high as 60 mm Hg. (**S/P**) Oral acetazolamide is likely used in most emergencies but should not be used for patients with advanced kidney disease, or other cases where there is marked depression of serum sodium or potassium levels. Acetazolamide should not be used in patients with a known history of allergic reactions to any similar chemical compounds such as the sulphonamide anti-infective drugs (used for urinary tract or bronchial infections, e.g. sulphamethoxazole). However, with current limited usage of sulphonamide drugs it is unlikely that a patient will be aware of such an allergy or potential cross-sensitivity.

(iii) intravenous acetazolamide. In very substantial cases of angle closure glaucoma, acetazolamide may be administered by intravenous infusion, by a physician in a hospital. A special vial containing 500 mg acetazolamide powder is reconstituted with 10 mL saline for injection *i.v.* and administered over a few minutes. The infusion should start to lower IOP within 15 minutes and the same contraindictions and limitations to use apply as for oral acetazolamide.

(iv) mannitol injections. Mannitol [*man-ee-tol*] is also an effective osmotic diuretic. Special solutions containing 10, 20, or 25 % mannitol solutions for intravenous infusion (e.g. PoM **Mannitol**, non-proprietary) may be used by a physician in the hospital emergency room as part of the management of the angle closure patient following referral. A typical dose would be 1 g / kg administered over several minutes, i.e. 300 mL of a 25 % solution. Mannitol is less likely to precipitate changes in glucose balance in the diabetic, unless the diabetes has progressed to a stage where kidney function is significantly impaired. The efficacy of these injections is very similar to oral glycerol but the procedure must be done in a hospital because of the risk of adverse effects of injecting such a relatively large volume of solution into the body over a relatively short time period.

(v) apraclonidine 1 % eyedrops. Apraclonidine [*a-prah-cloe-ni-deen*] (available as PoM **Iopidine**[R]) eyedrops are primarily indicated for use prior to ocular surgery for open angle glaucoma, e.g. an iridotomy or iridectomy. As such, these eye drops will either be used for a few days or weeks prior to surgery, or used just 1 hour prior to, and immediately following the procedure. The drug is not approved for use in the management of angle-closure glaucoma, where surgery is not being performed promptly. It can be noted however that some clinicians (primarily in the USA) have proposed that 2 *gtt* apraclonidine can be used as an adjunct to manage angle closure (presumably just prior to referral for surgery). Specific clinical trials or case histories do not appear to have been reported.

(vi) timolol [*tim-oh-lol*] 0.5 % eye drops. Controversial !. Acute dosing of the eye with timolol eye drops should lower IOP fairly rapidly. This procedure may be carried out with or without a miotic. However, the use of timolol eye drops (or any other *beta*-adrenergic-blocking drug) in such a manner is contraindicated in patients with any form of airways disease (asthma etc.), major cardiac disease and advanced diabetes. Suggested regimens range from q 30 min to as short as q 10 min, but there do not appear to be controlled studies published to show the safety or efficacy of this in cases of angle-closure, nor on the number of drops that would generally be required. This is not a generally approved indication for timolol eye drops.

NOTE on alcohol (ethanol, ethyl alcohol) and IOP. Alcohol (not methanol) can act as a powerful osmotic diuretic and thus lower IOP substantially. Its oral administration for this purpose is <u>not</u> a standard medical procedure. However, rapid consumption of two or more measures of high proof whisky (or its equivalent) should start to lower IOP (even from 50 or 60 mm Hg) some 15 to 30 min later; additional measures could even be administered if the effect was not considered adequate. Even though it could be the only "medication" available in a remote area, the substantial side effects associated its administration should not be overlooked, including the suitability of the patient for subsequent admission to an emergency room at a later point in time.

After an angle-closure has been managed in the short term, a patient will likely be referred for laser treatment, e.g. a laser iridotomy that will allow a continuous flow of aqueous humour through the iris tissue to prevent its accumulation under the iris after any pupillary block (that would result in recurrence of the angle closure).

OVERVIEW OF SYSTEMIC DRUG INTERACTIONS WITH THE ANTERIOR SEGMENT OF THE EYE

*Purpose of chapte*r. Systemically-administered drugs can reach the eye muscles via the general systemic circulation or via secretory sites within or around the eye and can affect the position or movement of the eye or the muscles inside the eye. Since any use of diagnostic or therapeutic drugs on the eye requires consideration of any side effects of systemic medications, this chapter provides an overview will be provided of systemic drug interactions with the extra-ocular muscles, the eyelids, pupil, ciliary body, lacrimal system conjunctiva and cornea.

1. DYSFUNCTION of the COORDINATED ACTIVITY OF THE EXTRAOCULAR MUSCLES (including EYEBLINK ACTIVITY).

MIMS and the BNF list a range of adverse reactions related to the function of the extra-ocular muscles. Descriptions such as visual disturbances, CNS disturbances, extra-pyramidal reactions, or involuntary motor activities should all be taken as indicators of possible disturbances in binocular vision, in addition to the well recognized descriptors such as blurred vision, diplopia and nystagmus. The magnitude of the effects that can be reported or observed are very dependent upon when the medications were taken and the effects should subside once the medication is discontinued.

Common examples include use of benzodiazepines such as nitrazepam (e.g. PoM **Mogadon**[R]), various anti-epilepsy drugs (although some of the effects may be more due to the involuntary muscle activity associated with epilepsy itself) such as phenytoin (e.g. PoM **Epanutin**[R]; especially in children), gabapentin (e.g PoM **Neurontin**[R]), or carbamazepine (e.g. PoM **Tegretol**[R]), phenothiazines such as chlorpromazine (e.g. PoM **Largactil**[R]) with patients general condition also perhaps resulting in abnormal eye movements / eye blinking. Doses of alcohol above the legal limit can affect binocular vision.

2. PALPEBRAL APERTURE (EYELID POSITION)

A number of drugs can affect the eyelid muscles to produce either a mild ptosis (usually transient or periodic) or slight widening of palpebral aperture. The impact of such a ptosis can range from a heavy lid sensation, Widening of the palpebral aperture may be of consequence for RGP contact lens wear, or in borderline cases of inadequate lid closure.

Drugs reported to cause ptosis include barbiturates, benzodiazepines (e.g. nitrazepam, PoM **Mogadon**[R]), select anti-arthritis drugs (e.g. hydroxy-chloroquine; PoM **Plaquenil**[R]; penicillamine; PoM **Pendramine**[R]), and high doses of alcohol. The ptosis may be described as a myasthenic condition. Widening of palpebral aperture can follow use of indirect-acting adrenergics or serotoninergics used for medicinal purposes (e.g. MAO inhibitors such as phenelzine, PoM **Nardil**[R]) or recreational purposes (e.g. amphetamines, cocaine, etc.).

3. PUPIL DILATION (MYDRIASIS)

A large number of systemic medications with cholinergic blocking effects have "glaucoma" listed as either a **C/I** or **S/P** because cases of a fixed dilated pupil and angle-closure have been reported for patients taking these drugs. Indirect-acting adrenergic drugs can still cause mydriasis but pose lower risks for angle-closure (including that via pupil block) if the pupil still retains some light reactivity. Patient management includes providing screening of susceptible individuals for narrow-angles (as well as generally considering whether systemic medications could change the anterior chamber angle in any patient), and identifying patients with a history of intermittent angle-closure to permit timely referral of patients back to the prescriber of the medications. Patient counselling is appropriate for use of any P Medicines in relation to the effects of mydriasis (glare, photophobia), the anterior chamber angle and "glaucoma".

Mydriasis can be caused by cholinergic blockers (atropine-like drugs) being used for stomach or GI tract ailments, nausea, motion sickness, irritable bowel syndrome or urinary incontinence (e.g. dicyclomine, PoM **Merbentyl**[R]; hyoscine, P / PoM **Buscopan**[R] or P **Kwells**[R]; skin patches containing hyoscine [scopolamine], PoM **Scopoderm-TTS**[R]; oxybutynin, P/ PoM **Ditropan**[R], PoM **Cystrin**[R] or PoM **Oxybutynin**, generic; tolterodine, PoM **Detrusitol**[R]; propiverine, PoM **Detrunorm**[R]), selective cholinergic blockers such as ipratropium (e.g Rx **Atrovent**[R], PoM **Respontin**[R], PoM **Rinatec**[R]), systemic drugs that have cholinergic-blocking side effects (e.g. disopyramide, PoM **Rythmodan**[R]; phenothiazines such as chlorpromazine, PoM **Largactil**[R], or prochlorperazine, PoM **Stemetil**[R]), tricyclic antidepressants (e.g. trimipramine, PoM **Surmontil**[R], or amitriptyline, PoM **Tryptizol**[R]) and older sedating (H_1-blocking) anti-histamines (e.g. bromopheniramine P **Dimotane**[R], chlorpheniramine, P **Piriton**[R]), indirect adrenergics or indirect serotoninergics including SNRI's (e.g. venlafaxine; PoM **Efexor**[R]), NARI's (e.g. reboxetine, PoM **Edronax**[R]), NaSSA's (e.g. mirtazapine; PoM **Zispin**[R]), MAO inhibitors (e.g. phenelzine; PoM **Nardil**[R]), RIMA's (e.g. moclobemide; PoM **Manerix**[R]), SSRI's (e.g. fluoxetine, PoM **Prozac**[R]; and fluvoxamine, PoM **Luvox**[R]) or other medicines with indirect-acting adrenergic effects include dexamphetamine (CD **Dexedrine**[R]) and methylphenidate (CD **Ritalin**[R]). The overuse (abuse) of direct-acting adrenergics found in dilute solutions of xylometazoline (P **Otrivin**[R] Nasal Drops) can also precipitate angle closure.

4. PUPILLARY MIOSIS

Miosis, with loss of light and near-point reflexes, is a noticeable characteristic of high doses of narcotic analgesics such as morphine, especially if administered *i.v.*; these are pinpoint pupils (1.5 mm). Other systemic drugs can produce a lesser miosis such as morphine-related drugs (e.g. pethidine, CD **Pethidine**[R]; buprenorphine, CD **Temgesic**[R]), CNS sedatives (e.g. alcohol or clonidine; PoM **Catapres**[R]), or oral cholinergic drugs (e.g. bethanechol, PoM **Myotonine**[R]; pilocarpine, Rx **Salagen**[R]), or adrenergic blockinging drugs such as indoramin (PoM **Doralese**[R]).

6. CYCLOPLEGIA

Most systemically-administered drugs that cause mydriasis can also interact with the ciliary body to relax it and cause a relative cycloplegic state; the patient is likely to report blurred vision if of a susceptible age. Any assessment of refractive error and / or true spectacle needs should be postponed until the medications are reduced or discontinued. Those systemically-administered drugs with the potential to cause cycloplegia include any atropine-like drug or those with cholinergic blocking side effects, repeated doses of histamine H_1-blocking drugs (bromopheniramine etc.), tricyclic anti-depressants (trimipramine etc.), MAO inhibitors (phenelzine etc.) and even SSRI's (fluoxetine etc.).

7. PSEUDOMYOPIA

A drug-induced pseudomyopia is the term given to an involuntary over-accommodation (and myopic shift) that results from a drug-induced contraction of the ciliary body.

Pseudomyopia can be caused by morphine-related drugs (e.g. pethidine, buprenorphine), CNS sedatives (e.g. alcohol or clonidine), oral cholinergic drugs (e.g. bethanechol, pilocarpine), oral adrenergic blocking drugs such as indoramin, oral anti-histamines (H_2-blocking drugs, e.g. cimetidine [*sigh-meh-ti-deen*]; P/PoM **Tagamet**[R]), tetracycline antibiotics (e.g. minocycline, PoM **Minocin**[R]), sulphonamide anti-infectives (e.g. sulphamethoxazole), carbonic anhydrase inhibitors (e.g. acetazolamide), cardiac glycosides (e.g. digoxin [*dye-jox-inn*]; PoM **Lanoxin**[R]). If significant miosis accompanies the pseudomyopia, then the patient is at (low) risk for pupil block.

8. LACRIMAL SYSTEM and TEAR FILM.

A certain quantity of lacrimal secretion is required to maintain a normal tear film. The balance between secretion, evaporation and tear film drainage will be different for each patient so the effects are relative only. Systemic drug interactions with the tear film can be classified into hyposecretion, hypersecretion and changes in tear film quality. Management of any tear film deficiency requires the use of simple artificial tears, and even ocular lubricants in more extreme cases, while hypersecretion may produce a 'wet dry eye'.

Lacrimal hyposecretion is that which is lower than that required to maintain a stable tear film volume leading to susceptibility to ocular irritation, reduced tolerance to contact lenses. The effect can be produced by oral diuretics, especially thiazide diuretics (e.g. hydrochlorothiazide, PoM **HydroSaluric**[R]), cholinergic blockers (atropine-like drugs) being used for stomach or GI tract ailments, nausea, motion sickness, irritable bowel syndrome or urinary incontinence (e.g. dicyclomine, PoM **Merbentyl**[R]; hyoscine, P / PoM **Buscopan**[R] or P **Kwells**[R]; skin patches containing hyoscine [scopolamine] PoM **Scopoderm-TTS**[R]; oxybutynin, P/ PoM **Ditropan**[R], PoM **Cystrin**[R] or PoM **Oxybutynin**, generic; tolterodine, PoM **Detrusitol**[R]; propiverine, PoM **Detrunorm**[R]), selective cholinergic blockers such as ipratropium (e.g PoM **Atrovent**[R], PoM **Respontin**[R], PoM **Rinatec**[R]), drugs that have cholinergic-blocking side effects (e.g. disopyramide, PoM **Rythmodan**[R]; phenothiazines (e.g. chlorpromazine, PoM **Largactil**[R], or prochlorperazine, PoM **Stemetil**[R]), tricyclic antidepressants (e.g. trimipramine, PoM **Surmontil**[R], or amitriptyline, PoM **Tryptizol**[R]) and older sedating (H_1-blocking) anti-histamines (e.g. bromopheniramine P **Dimotane**[R], chlorpheniramine, P **Piriton**[R]). Benzodiazepines (e.g. oral nitrazepam, PoM **Mogadon**[R]) and phenothiazines (e.g. oral chlorpromazine, PoM **Largactil**[R] or prochlorperazine, PoM **Stemetil**[R]) can also disturb normal lid-tear film interactions (including spontaneous eye-blink characteristics) leading to a destabilised tear film. Some *beta*-adrenergic blocking drugs (e.g. oral propranolol, PoM **Inderal**[R]; atenolol (PoM **Tenormin**[R]) can reduce lacrimal secretion but only some patients are really sensitive. This type of effect should be carefully distinguished from a severe type IV auto-immune, adverse drug reaction (the oculomuco-cutaneous syndrome) seen to a once-marketed (now withdrawn) oral *beta*-adrenergic blocker, practolol. Other anti-hypertension drugs can cause an irritative conjunctivitis, e.g. oral *alpha*$_1$ adrenergic blockers (e.g. prazosin, PoM **Hypovase**[R]) or *alpha*$_2$-adrenergics (e.g. oral clonidine; PoM **Catapres**[R]). Changes in tear film quality (leading to dry eye symptoms) may be seen following use of older and modern oral contraceptives and with use of hormone replacement therapy (HRT).

In contrast, lacrimal <u>hypersecretion</u>, which may only be the indirect result of suboptimal lacrimal drainage, can be caused by excessive use of topical nasal decongestants such as xylometazoline (e.g. P **Otrivin**[R] Nasal Drops) as a result of a "rebound effect" that causes hypersecretion. The use of narcotic analgesics, direct-acting cholinergics (e.g. oral pilocarpine, PoM **Salagen**[R]), indirect-acting cholinergics (e.g. pyridostigmine, PoM **Mestinon**[R]; donepezil, PoM **Aricept**[R]) could also promote lacrimal secretion that could actually be beneficial. However, anti-cancer medications can produce a general toxic reaction to the conjunctiva as well as chronic hypersecretion (e.g. oral cytarabine, PoM **Cytosar**[R]).

9. PERI-OCULAR SKIN and EYELID MARGINS

Changes in <u>pigmentation</u> intensity and / or uniformity on eyelids result from *photosensitivity* reactions with use of tetracycline antibiotics (e.g.minocycline, PoM **Minocin**[R]), phenothiazines (e.g. chlorpromazine, PoM **Largactil**[R]), and amiodarone [*a-mee-oh-dar-one*; PoM **Cordarone-X**[R] and are essentially a cosmetic problem. Some ocular irritation can occur however, but this swelling of the lid margins is generally less than that which can result from lacrimal gland dysfunction or conjunctival changes seen with use of oral isotretinoin [*eye-soe-tre-ti-noyn*, PoM **Roaccutane**[R]] or anti-cancer medications (e.g. oral cytarabine, PoM **Cytosar**[R]).

10. CONJUNCTIVA

Pigmentary changes or deposits in the conjunctival epithelia are generally cosmetic changes, but may cause irritation and discomfort, especially if the drugs are of the type that might cause lacrimal hypersecretion (see above). Pigmentation, visible across the white of the eye and within the normal palpebral aperture also result from photosensitisation as caused by tetracycline antibiotics (e.g. minocycline, PoM **Minocin**[R]), phenothiazines (e.g. chlorpromazine, PoM **Largactil**[R]) or anti-epilepsy drugs (e.g. carbamazepine, PoM **Tegretol**[R]). The pigmentation may be associated with small conjunctival cysts. Such cosmetic changes need to be distinguished from conjunctival irritation associated with tear film deficiencies where the management requires counselling and the adjunct use of simple artificial tears, e.g. with use of oral isotretinoin (PoM **Roaccutane**[R]), anti-cancer medications (e.g. oral cytarabine, PoM **Cytosar**[R]), *alpha*$_1$ adrenergic blockers (e.g. prazosin, PoM **Hypovase**[R]) or *alpha*$_2$-adrenergics (e.g. oral clonidine; PoM **Catapres**[R]), possibly *beta*-adrenergic blocking drugs (e.g. oral propranolol; PoM **Inderal**[R]) and diuretics (e.g. hydrochlorothiazide, PoM **HydroSaluric**[R]). Conjunctivitis has also been reported following use of modern as well as older oral contraceptives, and with use of hormone replacement therapy (HRT).

11. CORNEA

Photosensitisation of the cornea can produce deposits in the corneal epithelium (and perhaps the posterior corneal stroma and the corneal endothelium) which form whorl-like or broken pattern deposits. These have been reported after use of amiodarone (PoM **Cordarone-X**[R]), flecainide (PoM **Tambocor**[R]), chloroquine (PoM **Avloclor**[R], PoM **Nivaquine**[R]), hydroxychloroquine (PoM **Plaquenil**[R]), tamoxifen [*tam-ox-ee-fen*, PoM **Tamofen**[R]), some NSAID's such as indomethacin (PoM **Indocid**[R]) and naproxen (PoM **Naprosyn**[R]). Refractile deposits in the epithelium, without any obvious pattern being present, can occur with use of gold salts (e.g. auranofin, PoM **Ridaura**[R]) , while dust-like deposits can form after use of phenothiazines (e.g. chlorpromazine, PoM **Largactil**[R]) or certain anti-epilepsy drugs (e.g. carbamazepine, PoM **Tegretol**[R]). The management of corneal deposits is usually uncomplicated. If corneal deposits develop, then these deposits on their own are not a reason for discontinuing the medication but if a significant reduction (e.g. 2 lines) in visual acuity developed, then referral is advisable. The use of some of the drugs may also cause changes in the tear film and then produce mild symptoms (which can be managed with simple artificial tears). In rare cases, epithelial and even general corneal oedema can develop. The deposits may slowly resolve over 3 to 9 months when the drugs are discontinued.

The potential adverse reactions, and commonly used terms, are provided in the summary table on the next page.

Table 1: SUMMARY of POSSIBLE ADVERSE EFFECTS OF SYSTEMIC MEDICATIONS ON THE ANTERIOR SEGMENT

SITE OF EFFECT	TYPE OF EFFECT	drugs
EOM's	nystagmus dipolopia	nitrazepam, phenytoin, gabapentin, carbamazepine, chlorpromazine, alcohol
PALPEBRAL APERTURE	ptosis	barbiturates, nitrazepam, penicillamine hydroxychloroquine, alcohol
	widening	phenelzine, amphetamines, cocaine
PUPIL	mydriasis photophobia	dicyclomine, hyoscine (scopolamine), tolterodine, propiverine, oxybutynin, disopyramide, chlorpromazine, prochlorperazine, trimipramine, amitriptyline, bromo / chlorpheniramine, venlafaxine, mirtazapine, phenelzine, moclobemide, fluoxetine, fluvoxamine, dexamphetamine, methylphenidate, xylometazoline
	miosis	morphine, pethidine, alcohol, clonidine, bethanechol, pilocarpine
ACCOMODATION	cycloplegia	see mydriasis
	pseudomyopia	see miosis and cimetidine, minocycline, sulphamethoxazole, acetazolamide, digoxin
LACRIMAL GLANDS	dry eyes	hydrochlorthiazide, dicyclomine, hyoscine (scopolamine), tolterodine, propiverine, oxybutynin, belladonna alkaloids, disopyramide, chlorpromazine, trimipramine, amitriptyline, bromo / chlorpheniramine, nitrazepam, propranolol, atenolol, prazosin, clonidine
	epiphora	xylometazoline, chlorpheniramine, morphine, pethidine, pilocarpine, pyridostigmine, donepezil, cytarabine
EYELIDS	pigmentation	minocycline, chlorpromazine, amiodarone
	irritation	isotretinoin, cytarabine
CONJUNCTIVA	pigmentation	minocycline, chlorpromazine, carbamazepine
	conjunctivitis	isotretinoin, cytarabine, prazosin, clonidine, propranolol, hydrochlorthiazide, oral contraceptives, HRT
CORNEA	deposits	amiodarone, flecainide, hydroxychloroquine, chloroquine, tamoxifen, indomethacin, naproxen, gold salts, chlorpromazine, carbamazepine

A much more extensive coverage of this topic can be found in "**General Pharmacology for Primary Eye Care**" (Doughty) wherein ADR's are discussed within the fuller context of use of the medications.

RE-WETTING SOLUTIONS, MOISTURISERS, ARTIFICIAL TEARS, and OCULAR LUBRICANTS

Purpose of chapter. There are usually a number of preparations available for what are referred to as tear deficiencies, whether this be naturally occurring or that result from the use of systemic medications. Some of these solutions are specifically labelled for use as "re-wetting drops" (and may actually be listed as medical devices with a 'C ' symbol) while the rest may be referred to as artificial tears, moisturisers or ocular lubricants. The media and press can sometimes be saturated with advertisements for these products. It is the goal of this chapter to make some sense of these products and to provide practical guidelines for their use.

1. CONTACT LENS RE-WETTING SOLUTIONS

A number of products are usually available which are specifically designated for re-wetting a contact lens while in place on the eye. These products are labelled as 're-wetting drops' and / or 'comfort drops'. The current regulations on these solutions is such that they are not considered as pharmaceuticals and are marked with the 'C ' symbol. Their use is '*p.r.n.*', but from a clinical perspective one surely needs to question whether a patient should stay in contact lens wear if the perceived need for use of a re-wetting solution was more frequent than *q* 1 h.

The labelling of contact lens re-wetting solutions appears to be rather inconsistent but they generally contain saline, a polymer (usually a cellulose polymer) and probably a re-wetting agent (e.g. poloxamer or polyoxyl stearate). Multi-use bottles will contain a preservative. The solutions will likely contain a buffering agent (e.g. borate or citrate). Current products include a range of multi-use and unit dose products: -

(i) **Clerz**[R] **Comforting Eye Drops**. 10 mL bottles with NaCl, hydroxyethylcellulose and poloxamer 406, and preserved with sorbic acid 0.1 % / EDTA.

(ii) (Bauusch & Lomb) **Rewetting Drops**. 10 mL bottles with NaCl, hydroxypropylmethylcellulose and a wetting agent. Preserved with sorbic acid 0.25 %/ EDTA.

(iii) **Opti-Free**[R] **Rewetting Drops**. 15 mL bottles with NaCl and preserved with polidronium chloride / EDTA.

(iv) **Revive**[R] **Comforting Eye Drops**. Unit dose containing NaCl and carboxymethylcellulose.

(v) **Lens Fresh**[R] **Comfort and Rewetting Drops**. Unit dose containing NaCl, polyethylene glycol 300 BP and polyoxyl 40 stearate.

(vi) **Artelac**[R] **SDU**. Unit dose containing hypromellose 0.32 %, and sorbitol.

(vii) **VisMed**[R]. Unit dose containing a balanced salts mixture and sodium hyaluronate 0.1 %. Another product (**Vislube**™) was available as an import before VisMed was available in the UK.

2. MOISTURISERS

Current regulations permit the marketing of a range of other eyedrops as non-medicinal, cosmetic products. These are being termed moisturisers or "aquafiers" and are marketed as providing soothing and refreshing effects for tired eyes etc. They should not be considered as true replacements for tear deficiency, for which artificial tears should be used. Nonetheless, the use of terms such as lubrication are likely to be found associated with the products. Guidelines for these use are essentially 'as needed' for temporary relief of ocular discomfort. They should not be used whilst or shortly before contact lens wear and their continuous use should be monitored (in case the patient needs artificial tears).

(i) **Vital Eyes Moisturiser** (10 mL bottle, contains hydroxymethylpropyl cellulose 0.4 %) is an off-the-shelf product, that also contains vitamin A and vitamin E but (for which no medicinal claims are made).

(ii) **Rhoto Zi for Eyes** (7 mL bottle) contains povidone and poloxamer. It also contains d-camphor, for which no medicinal claims are made. It was originally introduced as an off-the-shelf, cosmetic product.

3. ARTIFICAL TEARS

Artificial tears (which is the label found on a number of ophthalmic products) can be considered either as simple or complex. The former category is simply meant to indicate that the eye drop contains some salts and usually one or two polymers in an aqueous vehicle. The latter category is used to indicate that the pharmaceutical contains high concentrations of special polymers or some other special ingredients (that a practitioner or patient may wish to consider). Complex artificial tears are usually more expensive than simple artificial tears, even if for multiple use. Some of the simple artificial tears products may also be called "ocular lubricants" but contain only low concentrations of the polymers; these should be considered as distinct from true lubricants.

Simple artificial tears are formulated so that their physico-chemical properties are either similar to the normal tears or at least readily miscible with and compatible with human tears. Artificial tears are generally isotonic or slightly hypotonic to the tear film, i.e. have an osmolality of c. 250 to 300 mOsm/kg. Artificial tears generally have a pH that is slightly acid to "normal" tears, i.e. have a pH between 6.5 and 7.5. Simple artificial tear products generally have a viscosity that is similar to, or slightly increased above that expected for human tears; this is achieved with low concentrations of various polymers. More complex artificial tears contain two polymers. Common examples of polymers include cellulose polymers [e.g. carboxymethylcellulose (CMC), hydroxyethylcellulose (HEC), or hypromellose (also known as hydroxypropylmethylcellulose; (HPMC)], polyvinyl alcohol (PVA), polyethylene glycol (e.g. PEG400), polyvinyl-pyrrolidone (also known as povidone or polyvidone). Other polymers include polysorbate 40 or 80 (TWEEN[R] 80 etc.), carbowax 40 or 80, carbomer 940 (polyacrylic acid), or poloxamer 40 or 188 etc., dextran 70 etc. The number after the polymer name provides an indication of the molecular size of the polymer. Some of these polymers may impart considerable viscosity to these solutions; at the higher levels, these should be considered as true lubricants (see below). The overall osmolality (tonicity) and pH specifications are achieved with salts and buffers and small quantities of NaOH or HCl; some or all of these details may be provided on the product label.

For the clinical use of simple or complex artificial tears, a number of things should be considered : -

(**a**) objective assessments. Before suggesting, or advocating, the use of either artificial tears and /or ocular lubricants, consideration should be given to what objective evaluation of the tear film and ocular surface can be done; this can include using dyes / stains. With such a move, even if the results are not very convincing (as they can be in many borderline patients), they provide at least a semi-quantitative assessment rather than just relying on symptomatology or gross and often ambiguous external signs.

(**b**) establish true baseline condition. It may be very useful to get a symptomatic patient to discontinue use of any ophthalmic products they are currently using for at least a day before a detailed eye examination. Knowing the true nature of a patients condition can be most helpful in deciding on which artificial tear products to use.

(**c**) patient preferences. Patient comfort with and ease of use of products of artificial tears is important if they are going to be compliant with a recommended regimen. Some artificial tears sting; some don't. Some artificial tears have a distinct odour and / or "taste funny" following drainage through the naso-lacrimal duct; others don't. Some artificial tears are in very small bottles; others are in bigger bottles etc. Consider patient dexterity in being able to handle small vs. large bottles as well.

(**d**) preserved or non-preserved artificial tears ?. Some patients may need preservative-free artificial tears. A few patients may develop allergy to a preservative in artificial tears. While thimerosal and methylparabens / propylparabens may be more active in this respect, these can occur to benzalkonium chloride as well. Unit-dose and other preservative-free products are available, but there really is not any justification in starting a patient on these products (or continuing with them) unless there are clear indications of adverse reactions to the drops or the patient thinks that they need the drops at least 6 X day.

(**e**) general allergy to eye drops ? (**C/I**). Patient sensitization to any of the ingredients of a pharmaceutical is a reason not to use such products; even for artificial tear use, patients should still be advised to discontinue if any irritation, etc. develops. For every pharmaceutical, every reasonable effort must be made to establish whether or not the patient is hypersensitive to the drug or any of the other ingredients and this can only be effectively done through appropriate questions being asked each time (even though some might argue that these are "only artificial tears").

If significant ocular discomfort or signs persist or develop; artificial tear product use should be promptly discontinued and an eye examination arranged. Equally importantly, it should be assessed whether there has been over-use of these products, since this can occur if a patient feels they need artificial tears very frequently (i.e. q 1h or more often). In these cases, the appropriate management involves the use of lubricants or complex artificial tear products and / or consideration for further lacrimal or lacrimal duct assessment (including consideration of punctal plugs to retain the tears). No artificial tear can be expected to effectively compete with an ongoing disease process (e.g. mild infection etc.) or display satisfactory efficacy if there is poor ocular and periocular hygiene; always check and advise accordingly.

(**e**) cost ?. Consider the cost of artificial tears to patients. Simpler products tend to cost less than complex products and if a patient can be adequately managed on a simple artificial tear, why spend more ?. Unit dose formulations are generally much more expensive than multi-use bottles; larger bottles (i.e. 10 to 15 mL) tend to be cheaper than small bottles (i.e. those of 2 to 5 mL).

The various products are all similar in terms of affording comfort so allowing for patient preferences in selection (see earlier). Confidence in products can be gained by largely using only one or two products for most patients. This is a reasonable approach to considering which products to keep a stock of, or routinely recommend to patients. It is clearly impossible to stock all of the many different artificial tear products in a regular optometric practice. Other artificial tear products can then be tried if a preferred product does not produce the desired results, or elicits a discomfort reaction from one or more patients.

(**f**) choosing a regimen for use of simple artificial tears. For the most part, simple artificial tears are for occasional use (i.e. *p.r.n*) for the relief of mild and uncomplicated symptoms. These may arise from working for extended periods in an atmosphere that irritates the eyes, from inadequate blinking (due to over-work or general tiredness), to a dry atmosphere, etc. For such cases, the artificial tear is thus little more than a mini-bottle of eyewash since the one to two drops that are instilled can be expected to simply wash out the existing tear film, and remove debris and irritants.

In many cases, occasional use of simple artificial tears is all that is required to obtain relief from symptoms. It can be most useful however to place a patient on a specific regimen (e.g. *q.d.s.*) for the use of a product. This regimen should also be for a finite period of time (e.g. 1 to 4 weeks) and then reassess if this regimen works. This places part of the decision making on the optometrist rather than simply leaving everything to the patient. In the extreme, providing, no discomfort is associated with the use of the artificial tears, most products that fall into this general category can be used *p.r.n.* or literally "as often as required" (a statement on some product labels). However such use does not mean that the patient is getting the optimum treatment. A fixed period of monitored treatment can make all the difference between effective relief from symptoms and perpetual discomfort.

(**g**) patient education and communication. Compliance with suggested therapy can be expected to be better if there is education and communication; this is the opposite of assuming "intelligence" (common sense) and just handing out eye drops with a silent "use these". In chronic and or more severe cases of irritation and discomfort, better management is likely achieved if the patient is examined objectively before and after the use of the artificial tear products, especially if a patient presents with current symptoms. This also provides an excellent opportunity to discuss instillation technique and care of the artificial tear products with patients.

CURRENT ARTIFICIAL TEARS and RELATED PRODUCTS
Examples of some currently available products for management of uncomplicated dry eye symptoms include the following -

(a) saline eyedrops without polymers to enhance viscosity, e.g. P **Sodium chloride eyedrops** (generic, 15 mL bottles), also known as Normal Saline eye drops.

(b) hypromellose polymers at 0.3 % (e.g. P **Moisture Eyes** or several generics as P **Hypromellose** 0.3 %, 10 mL bottles) or with dextran 70 0.1 % (e.g. P **Tears Naturale**[R]; 15 mL bottle). P **Optrex**[R] **Dry Eye Therapy Eye Drops** (10 mL bottle) was discontinued in early 1998.

(c) with hypromellose 0.5 %, e.g. P **Isopto Plain**[R] (10 mL bottle).

(d) with polyvinyl alcohol (PVA) 1.4 % as the polymer, e.g. P **Liquifilm Tears**[R] (15 mL bottles); P **Sno Tears**[R] (10 mL bottle).

(e) with a slightly lower PVA (1 %) content and slightly hypotonic vehicle, e.g. P **Hypotears**[R] (10 mL bottle).

All these multi-use bottles products (above) contain preservatives, usually benzalkonium chloride. The following are preservative-free :-

(f) unit dose **Minims**[R] **Sodium chloride** eye drops, containing 0.9 % NaCl are also available, as well as generic equivalents.

(g) SL **Artelac**[R] **SDU**. Unit dose containing hypromellose 0.32 %.

(h) P **Minims**[R] **Artificial Tears**, with hydroxyethylcellulose 0.44 %

(i) SL **Vital Eyes**[R]., with hydroxymethylpropyl cellulose 0.4 %.

(j) with polyvinyl alcohol 1.4 %, unit dose and preservative-free, e.g. P **Liquifilm Tears**[R] **Preservative Free**

(k) with polyvinyl alcohol and povidone, P **Refresh**[R], unit dose and preservative-free. Supply has been interrupted at times.

(l) with polyvidone 5 %, P **Oculotect**[R], unit dose and preservative-free.

4. OCULAR LUBRICANTS and OTHER PREPARATIONS.

The term ocular lubricant is a poor one for it is likely that any eye drops will provide some lubricating action and thus brief relief of symptoms for patients with really dry eyes. There appear to be few guidelines as to what might distinguish one product from another in terms of real lubricating efficacy and thus whether a product can be called an ocular lubricant or not. One approach is to accept that all products actually marketed as 'artificial tears' will provide some lubricating effects, but only those products designated with higher concentrations of polymers or special polymers, or mineral oil or petrolatum-based ingredients would be labelled as true lubricants. Some of these products will also fit under the category of 'complex' artificial tears in these sense that the formulation is complex.

(**S/P**) Some limitations do apply to the use of true ocular lubricants (beyond allergy to any of the ingredients): -

(**a**) lubricants are NOT for use as a primary therapy in cases of follicular conjunctivitis, especially where there is evidence to suggest *Chlamydia* infection. Managing the infection with antibiotics (e.g. oral tetracycline antibiotics or other antibiotics such as azithromycin) should be the primary goal, and such patients should be referred to special STD clinics at the hospital etc.

(**b**) lubricants should be used cautiously in cases of toxic keratitis produced by chronic use of ophthalmic pharmaceuticals or systemic medications. Discontinuation of the therapy causing the toxic reaction should be the primary goal rather than simply using the lubricant to cover up the symptoms and signs.

(**c**) lubricants should be used cautiously in cases of chronic irritation of a vernal / atopic type precipitated by a poor working environment or other irritant. Protection of the eyes from the irritant or systemic therapy to · manage the atopic disease may be required for effective management.

A lubricant, as opposed to simple artificial tears, is indicated for use whenever there is non-infective or non-toxic chronic irritation and inflammation of the conjunctiva that is accompanied by poor traction of the lids across the ocular surface, i.e. a patient with chronic dry eye conditions such as keratoconjunctivitis sicca (Sjogrens syndrome). A true lubricant, by definition, does not replace the tear film with a simple aqueous fluid but with a lubricating film with a long residency time at the ocular surface. The true lubricant thus cannot be expected to either improve the hydration of the dry ocular surface, nor relieve day-to-day scratchy and itchy symptoms. Therefore, supplementation of lubricant use with simple artificial tears may be very effective in some patients. The selection of a lubricant product depends upon how much friction one wishes to try to reduce and for how long. For example, nightly use of a lubricating ointment could mean a change in daily regimen from simple artificial tears q 1 h, to the use of lubricating tears q 2 h or q. 3 h, or a liquid gel q 4 h or q 6h. Ointments can be used during the day q 3 h but some patients may not like the slight "smeary vision" effects that may result for a brief period of time after the application of the ointment. Preservative-free or lanolin-free products are for patients who exhibit sensitivity to either of these ingredients.

The following can be considered as true ocular lubricants -

(i) cellulose polymer containing products at the 1 % level, e.g. hypromellose (P **Isopto Alkaline**[R] Eye-drops, 10 mL bottle), or CMC (**Celluvisc**[R], unit dose, available for special use on a named patient basis)

(ii) carbomer 940 0.2 %, e.g. P **Viscotears**[R] Liquid gel, 10 mL tube) or P **GelTears**[R], 5 mL and 10 mL tubes. These CARBOMER "eye-drops" (preserved with cetrimide) contain a special polyacrylic acid that, on mixing with the natural tear film, forms a viscous gel. Since the gel is somewhat acidic, it may produce some irritation but a longer ocular contact time is still expected, even in an irritated teary eye. Recommended for *t.d.s.* or *q.d.s.* use.

Sodium hyaluronate may also be available as a hospital-formulated bottle of eyedrops from sodium hyaluronate solution that is used for intra-ocular injection (PoM **Healonid**[R]). Unit-dose eye drops containing glycerol (glycerine) are marketed in the USA, and diluted glycerin(e) solutions (< 10 %) could also be formulated by a hospital pharmacy from sterile glycerin and water or saline. Solutions of methylcellulose 1 % may also be prepared for hospital use. Castor oil eye drops were once widely used whenever there was an emergency hospital admission for "something in the eye" on the logic that the substantial lubricating effects would help remove the foreign body and reduce the chance of substantial scratch damage to the ocular surface. Castor oil eye drops were once marketed (e.g. PoM **Minims**[R] **Castor oil**) and while no commercial products are currently available, these could still be used in hospitals, or a solution of light liquid paraffin used as eye drops.

(**iii**) lubricating ointments containing low quantities of liquid paraffin or mineral oil, <u>white</u> paraffin and low concentrations of wool fat derivatives and some form of lanolin, unless otherwise specifically stated otherwise (e.g. P **Lacri-lube**[R] Eye ointment in 3.5 g tubes; P **Lubri-Tears**[R] ophthalmic ointment, 5 g tubes).

(**iv**) <u>bland ointments</u> containing of a mixture of higher concentrations of <u>yellow</u> soft paraffin, lower concentrations of liquid paraffin with wool fat, e.g. P **Simple Eye Ointment** (generic, 3.5 g tube). Another ointment (P **Lubrifilm**[R] Eye ointment, 3.5 g tubes) was marketed, but its availability is currently uncertain.

(**v**) acetylcysteine eye-drops. This viscous solution of 5 % acetylcysteine in with hypromellose 0.35 % (e.g. PoM **Ilube**[R] Eye drops, 10 mL bottle) are used as lubricants with a cleansing action. The acetylcysteine is considered to be able to disperse abnormal mucous strands on the surface of the eyes of patients with severe disease, e.g. Sjogren's syndrome. The eye drops smell slightly sulphydrous and can elicit a marked stinging sensation lasting many minutes; the effect is more pronounced the higher concentration of acetylcysteine is. Such eye drops are best used under close supervision, and only for as long as needed to disperse filamentary mucous (usually only a day or so). Higher concentrations (up to 20 %) have been tried in various types of studies.

OPHTHALMIC TOPICAL DECONGESTANTS, TOPICAL ANTI-INFLAMMATORY DRUGS and ANTI-HISTAMINES.

Purpose of chapter. In some patients, the source of their ocular irritation and discomfort is a chemical irritant, an allergen or both together. For management of these conditions and to provide relief from symptoms, more than just simple artificial tears or eyewashes are needed since the vasodilation and mild inflammation has to treated. This is where topical ocular decongestants, topical ocular anti-histamines, topical ocular non-steroidal anti-inflammatory drugs and oral anti-histamines are used. In this chapter are details of these various types of products and why and how they are used to manage non-infectious irritation and allergic conjunctivitis.

1. TOPICAL DIRECT-ACTING DECONGESTANTS / non-prescription ANTI-HISTAMINES

These are available to the general public on request from a pharmacist, or may even be directly available through an optometrist. In UK-marketed products, at least four different decongestants are to be found in these products, sometimes on their own, or sometimes together in combination products. The decongestant activity is the result of direct *alpha*$_1$-adrenergic action or direct histamine H$_1$ blocking action. Both types of drugs will either attenuate vasodilatation, or even cause vasoconstriction (especially the adrenergics) - thus the term "decongestants". Most adrenergic drugs used in these products are considered to primarily interact with *alpha*$_1$ receptors on the blood vessels of the conjunctiva (to promote vasoconstriction). There is some evidence however that *alpha*$_2$ type receptors are also present in conjunctival tissue (including the blood vessels) and drug interaction with these receptors will help counter vasodilatation and also the other signs and symptoms of a mild inflammatory reaction. These other signs and symptoms include discomfort, puffiness / oedema (chemosis), reflex lacrimation, and all will probably be attenuated by use of the decongestant. If the products also contain an anti-histamine (H$_1$-blocking), additional efficacy against itchiness symptoms can be expected. All these products contain preservatives (usually benzalkonium chloride and edetate sodium).

(i) phenylephrine 0.12 % as an *alpha*$_1$-adrenergic in eye drops such as P **Isopto Frin**^{R} (10 mL bottle) with hypromellose and benzethonium chloride.

(ii) naphazoline *c.* 0.01 % as an *alpha*-adrenergic included in eye drops, and preserved with benzalkonium chloride, e.g. P **Murine**^{R}, 10 mL bottles. with benzalkonium chloride. Combination products containing naphazoline 0.01 % with astringents such as witch hazel 12 % (also known as *Hamamelis* water) are also available, e.g. P **Eye Dew**^{R} **Clear** or **Optrex Clearine**^{R}, 10 mL bottles.

(**iii**) naphazoline 0.01 % as an *alpha*-adrenergic with witch hazel 12.5 % (as an astringent) and brilliant blue dye (for cosmesis), and preserved with benzalkonium chloride, e.g. P **EyeDew**[R] **Blue**, 10 mL bottles.

(**iv**) xylometazoline 0.05 % as an adrenergic (with both $alpha_1$ and $alpha_2$ actions) in combination products with antazoline 0.5 % as a histamine H_1 blocker, and preserved with benzalkonium chloride and edetate sodium, e.g.P **Otrivine-Antistin**[R], 10 mL bottle.

A polymer is usually included in decongestant-containing products to promote ocular contact time. The relative concentrations of the polymers (viscosity agents) are different between products and thus the relative soothing / mild lubricant action of the products can be quite different between products. Some products are promoted as having longer-lasting effects, and in some cases this may simply be the result of the inclusion of one or more polymers into the eye drops.

GENERAL GUIDELINES FOR USE OF OCULAR DECONGESTANTS.

Eye whiteners can promptly relieve acute-onset symptoms, and greatly improve the cosmetic appearance of the external eye. For their effective clinical use, the following should be considered -

(**a**) all products are meant to provide occasional relief of symptoms associated with mildly-irritated eyes and to improve the cosmetic appearance of the external eye, eyelid margins, etc., e.g. use 2 to 3 times daily. All too often these reasons are reversed and the products are used to "whiten" eyes that really only need a good wash or even some sleep; *q* 2 h or > 6 X / day should be considered as excessive / over use. Overall however, these products are the "eye whiteners" and provide an effective means of self-medication to manage an eye with acute or sub-acute mild foreign body sensation, gritty feelings, etc., as well as the "pain across the front of my eyes" from a day in the sun, at the beach, pool, etc.

In evaluating patients, it should be remembered that the decongestants can be equally effective in promoting comfort and improving external signs. Therefore, before close examination of an irritated eye, adjust expectations of diagnoses and ratings accordingly. As a result of a very strong lay advertising as the "cure-all" for all types of irritated eyes, these products are frequently abused in the belief that they are effective as prophylactic as well as treatment drugs. The underlying risk in any patient who is using these products, even on just a daily basis, is that important signs and symptoms of an underlying disease are covered up. An equally important risk is that these products can be overused and a 'medicamentosa' (adverse reaction) results from a mild toxic reaction or type IV allergic reaction due to prior sensitisation to one of the ingredients, e.g. the active ingredient or a preservative. The means of sensitization can sometimes be systemic, e.g. a sensitivity to zinc sulphate (as found in P **Zinc Sulphate Eye-drops**, generic, used as astringents) could be associated with a systemic sensitivity to zinc oxide plasters, for example, while a preservative sensitivity could arise from prior eye make-up use.

(b) <u>the cause of the irritation should be identified</u>, rather than the eye drops being used indiscriminately, i.e. if there is a genuine allergic component, systemic anti-histamines would be appropriate (perhaps even as the primary medication). For dirt, dust, and irritating vapours, a good eyewash could achieve superior results !.

(c) the <u>efficacy of any of these products as prophylactic agents</u> is questionable. These types of products can reduce the ocular sensitivity to the agents that precipitate the cycle of hyperaemia / injection / mild oedema etc., (i.e. have slight prophylactic efficacy that is probably more related to slight reflex lacrimation functioning as a mini eye-wash). It has been advocated however that topical drug-induced vasoconstriction will reduce the severity of irritative conjunctivitis and the use of these products immediately before an anticipated exposure to a mild irritant or allergen may reduce the resultant severity of symptoms. Since many of these products sting a little on instillation, briefly stimulating tear flow can also prompt wash-out of irritants; water or a cold compress are also effective !.

(d) <u>excessive use of these products</u>, especially if there is continuing irritation (e.g. swimming pools, petrol vapours, dry eyes, etc.) can lead to a rebound effect in which the condition both becomes relatively refractory to the vasoconstrictive action of the decongestants and the vasculature re-dilates 4 to 6 h later to a greater level than before; symptoms do not necessarily get worse when the rebound signs appear.

SPECIFIC GUIDELINES FOR USE OCULAR DECONGESTANTS

(1) (**C/I**) The use of these products is contraindicated in narrow angle glau-coma; a listed **ADR** is angle closure. These products should therefore be only carefully recommended, or given to <u>elderly patients</u> if the IOP and / or anterior chamber angles are unknown. Since these are P Medicines, the products state "..should not be used by anyone with glaucoma".

(2) (**S/P**) for systemic diseases. These products should not be recom-mended / provided to any patient with substantial <u>blood pressure disor-ders</u>, any <u>cardiac disorders</u>, or a <u>history of stroke</u> or <u>hyperthyroidism</u> or if <u>pregnant</u>, i.e. treat these vasoconstrictors as if they were all phenyle-phrine. The concentration of the vasoconstrictors may be small but with over-use, systemic effects can occur. Many packaging or inserts for these products carry such warnings and may also list (labile) diabetes. It is not that these products contain high concentrations of dangerous drugs but simply that they can be so easily over-used so deliver a higher dose. The same types of precautions also apply to use of OTC nasal decongestants (e.g. P **Otrivine**[R] **Nasal Drops** or P **Sudafed**[R] nasal sprays containing oxymetazoline).

(3) (**INT**) (**S/P**) for concurrent medications. Use of these products should be carefully supervised in patients taking <u>MAO inhibitors</u> and related indirect-acting sympathomimetic or indirect-acting serotoninergic drugs; the risk is of systemic pressor effects (*cf.* phenylephrine 2.5 % eye drops). Product labels may only carry a statement concerning concurrent use of "anti-depressants" or in patients with depression (who are likely, at least periodically, to be medicated with anti-depressants).

COMMENTS for concurrent eye infections. These products should be avoided or their use limited for relief of symptoms in an eye with a known <u>infection</u>. This is the primary reason why most of these products carry a warning to the effect that they should not be used for people with "eye disease" while package inserts might say something to the effect that a "physician" should be consulted if irritation persists for more than a few days. For this reason, one should try to avoid (excessive) use of these products in young children who might have mild bacterial conjunctivitis.

NOTE on alternatives to topical ocular decongestants. Recently introduced are non-medicinal products that contain flower petal extracts (e.g. of lavender, orange flower and *Euphrasia*) as well as small quantities of witch hazel, and trace amounts of astringents (e.g. zinc sulphate 0.02 %) and decongestant (e.g. naphazoline 0.005 %). Such products (e.g. SL **Vital Eyes Brightener**) are designed to soothe tired / irritated eyes.

2. <u>TOPICAL OCULAR ANTI-HISTAMINES</u>

When an allergic component to chronic conjunctivitis is identified, the use of topical ocular anti-histamines is appropriate. Their use, on a repeated / chronic base is far preferable to the use of decongestants or non-prescription decongestant / antihistamine combinations because these products carry a lower risk of inducing sympathomimetic or other systemic side effects, i.e. there are few currently-listed limitations or contraindications to their use.

(i) levocabastine [*lee-voh-cab-as-teen*] 0.05 % eyedrops. This is available as both PoM **Livostin**^{R} (as a 4 mL bottle) and P **Livostin**^{TM} **Direct** (3 mL bottle). This H_1-blocking anti-histamine is being presented as having the ability to manage chronic conditions as effectively as mast cell stabilisers such as sodium cromoglycate (see later) but to be able to provide a faster onset achievement of a quiet eye, even to the extent of prompt relief of symptoms (because of its direct histamine-blocking action). Like other histamine H_1 blockers it will reduce vasodilatation. Since it is considered to have long-lasting actions, it can be used just *b.d.* as well as *t.d.s* or *q.d.s.* (depending on severity of the condition). Current UK recommendations are that a treatment period should not exceed 4 weeks in any one season. Not currently recommended for use in children below the age of 9 years (PoM product) or 12 years (P product). The P medicine product is licensed for seasonal allergic conjunctivitis only.

(ii) azelastine [*aye-zee-la'steen*] 0.05 % eye drops (PoM **Optilast**[R], as a 6 mL bottle). This H_1-blocking anti-histamine is also being presented as having the ability to manage chronic allergic eye conditions with prompt achievement of relief of symptoms (just as non-prescription anti-histamines and decongestants can) as it will reduce vasodilatation. As a result of high affinity binding (high potency) it can be used just *b.d.* as well as *t.d.s* or *q.d.s.* (depending on severity of the condition). No data is available on long term efficacy. Currently not recommended for use in children.

(iii) emedastine [*em-ay-da'steen*] is another H_1-blocking antihistamine also introduced in the UK in 1999 in eye drop form (as PoM **Emadine**[R], emedastine 0.05 %, 5 mL bottle). Intended for *b.d.s.* use, and recommended for patients as young as 3 years of age. Published data on clinical efficacy is however limited at this time.

(iv) olopatidine [*oh-la-pa-ti-deen*] is a new type of drug that is considered to have both direct histamine H_1-blocking actions and indirect histamine-blocking actions (to include "stabilisation" of mast cells). It was introduced, as eye drops, in the USA in 1997 (as PATANOL[TM]).

4. INDIRECT-ACTING TOPICAL OCULAR ANTI-INFLAMMATORY PREPARATIONS.

Some 10 to 15 % of the population have chronic symptomatic atopic diseases, with seasonal allergic conjunctivitis and irritative conjunctivitis being the most common of these diseases. Chronic ocular allergies, as with all inflammatory diseases of the external eye, can present with a wide spectrum of signs and symptoms. Decisions really need to be made, before instigating treatment, on the <u>severity</u> of the signs and symptoms and the <u>history</u> of these signs and symptoms, especially as to whether they are intermittent or sustained. Intermittent episodes of mild-to-moderate itching and lacrimation can usually be managed with eye-baths and decongestant / anti-histamine eye drops. However, a history of moderate-to-severe symptoms accompanied by mucoid discharge (often with nasal stuffiness etc.) is more likely to respond to a combination of repeated local therapy and systemic therapy. If there are simply persistent ocular signs (marked hyperaemia / injection) and symptoms (marked itching, lacrimation etc.), then chronic therapy with histamine-suppressant therapy is probably needed (i.e. with a group of drugs often referred to as mast cell stabilizers). Severe ocular involvement can include marked vasodilatation, chronic oedema of the lid margins and conjunctiva, along with infiltrates accompanied by a high level of discomfort / foreign body sensation. In such cases, any of the above treatment(s) <u>and</u> local or systemic corticosteroids and medications for the nasal and respiratory tract may also be necessary. Management of severe chronic cases is thus best effected by co-management with a general medical practitioner, as are paediatric cases.

MAST CELL STABILISERS

While widely used, "mast cell stabilisers" is a non-medical term of limited scientific use. The inadequacy of the term is simply because some or all of these drugs clearly do more than simply stabilise the mast cells. The overall result of treatment with these drugs is to reduce the release of histamine and other allergic reaction-producing chemicals and to reduce the reactions of the white blood cells to the allergens. Products with such indirect histamine-blocking actions include -

(**i**) sodium cromoglycate (alternatively known as disodium cromoglycate, cromolyn sodium, or cromolyn; will be renamed as sodium cromoglicate). The drug is a "mast cell stabiliser" with some actions on eosinophils and neutrophils as well. This drug is now widely available as a Pharmacy Medicine in 5 mL or 10 mL sizes as an ophthalmic solution at the 2 % concentration (e.g. P **Opticrom**[R] Allergy Eye Drops, P **Optrex Hayfever Allergy Eye Drops**[R], P **Hay-crom**[R] Hayfever Eye Drops, P **Clariteyes**[R] eye drops, and **Boots Hayfever Relief Allergy Eye Drops**. A P **Brol-Eze**[R] Eye Drops was marketed in 1997. All of the eye drops probably also contain benzalkonium chloride and edetate sodium. These P Medicines are available for general use by the public-at-large for management of seasonal allergic conjunctivitis and perennial allergic conjunctivitis.

Sodium cromoglycate 2 % eye drops are also available in larger 13.5 mL bottles. e.g. PoM **Opticron**[R] Eye Drops, PoM **Cusilyn**[R] Eye Drops, PoM **Hay-crom**[R] Eye Drops, PoM **Vividrin**[R] Eye Drops, PoM **Viz-On**[R] Eye Drops, and generic products. All of the eye drops probably also contain benzalkonium chloride and edetate sodium. The PoM products have a wider range of indications, including for VKC (see later).

Eye drops and ointment were once marketed at the 4 % concentration. An ophthalmic ointment (P/ PoM **Opticrom**[R], eye ointment, 5 g tube) was available until mid-1998, but was discontinued because of supply problems. The P product ointment was indicated for seasonal allergic conjunctivitis only, while the PoM product had wider uses (especially in patients who have difficulty with a *q.d.s.* regimen). Some stocks may still be available.

(**ii**) lodoxamide (also known as lodoxamide trometamol or lodoxamide tromethamine). A 0.1 % ophthalmic solution (PoM **Alomide**[R]; 10 mL bottle) is a "2nd generation" mast cell stabiliser, and now accepted as a dual-agent having substantial 'eosinophil inhibitor' activity. Such action in stressed regions of the conjunctival vasculature is considered to be of long term benefit in reducing infiltration / inflammation etc.

(**iii**) nedocromil sodium [*nee 'dock-roe-mill*] is available as eye drops (PoM **Rapitil**[R], 5 mL bottle). The solution has a distinctive canary yellow colour, and so definitely should not be used concurrently with soft contact lens wear. Indications for use are the same as for sodium cromoglycate.

GUIDELINES FOR USE OF MAST CELL STABILIZERS

These drugs are not "cure-all" products and their effective use requires consideration of the following -

(*i*) (**C/I**) Known sensitivity (allergy) to the drugs or any other ingredients of the pharmaceuticals. Cross-reactivity between mast cell stabilisers has not been reported, but should always be considered. To date, the number of allergic-type reactions for sodium cromoglycate products has been extraordinarily small, but it has yet to be established if the same record will be established for the other mast cell stabilisers.

(*ii*) (**IND**) mast cell stabilizers are indicated for prophylactic use to offset the severity of ocular reactions to allergens.

(*iii*) mast cell stabilizers are NOT indicated for provision of short term or acute relief; topical ocular decongestants, eye baths and cold compresses should do this. If such dramatic relief is provided to the patient (and some clinical studies have provided evidence that this type of effect can occur), one can argue that the patient did not really need these mast cell stabiliser drugs. There are two reason for this recommendation. One is simply one of cost in that even as P Medicines, bottles of these drugs usually cost more than 5 to 10 mL sized bottles of ocular decongestants or astringents. Secondly, eye drops containing sodium cromoglycate are not very stable and the bottle (including unused contents) should be discarded 1 month after opening.

(*iv*) dosing needs to be regular and continuous, e.g. *q* 4 h or *q* 6 h depending on severity of the condition, or the estimate of the allergen levels anticipated. Patients appear to be able to tolerate cromolyn sodium for extended periods of time (i.e. months) without there being significant reduction in the sensitivity to the drug or adverse reactions occurring; the same is currently assumed for lodoxamide eye drops. If a higher dosing (e.g. *q* 3 h) is considered necessary, then the patient should be advised that the recommended upper dosing limit is 16 drops day / eye. IF *q* 3 h dosing is not effective, supplementary medications are needed.

(*v*) patient education is important. The patient should be instructed that regular dosing is the only means by which these drugs can be expected to be effective and that it is important that they adhere to the dosing regimen that you recommend. The maintenance of a quiet eye throughout the day (in the presence of continuing allergen or irritants) may take 2 to 4 weeks of daily therapy to achieve for seasonal conjunctivitis, although some improvement can be expected in 7 to 10 days. For vernal conjunctivitis, 4 to 8 weeks of daily therapy may be required to achieve the maintenance state. Lodoxamide eye drops may produce effective stabilisation of the eye within 1 to 3 weeks, while nedocromil eye drops appear to be equivalent to sodium cromoglycate in terms of the type and extent of relief provided. For all three drugs, once the relatively quiet eye has been achieved, the therapy must be continued for as long as the allergen challenge or disease state persists.

(*vi*) only dispense (prescribe / recommend) <u>one bottle at a time</u>. The small bottle size (5 or 10mL) is designed to be used within 1 to 3 weeks and a practice of getting regular replacements from a pharmacy or prescription refills is generally superior (and recommended) to providing several bottles at one time. The same generally applies to the larger 13.5 mL PoM products. Such a plan of one-bottle-at-a-time allows for at least cursory check ups (to assess whether the eye drops are being used as recommended, and whether any irritation has developed from the use of the eye drops).

5. NON-STEROIDAL ANTI-INFLAMMATORY DRUGS

Other drugs have been developed for the management of seasonal and vernal conjunctivitis, but it is very important to note the current indications for use of products containing these drugs in the UK. Some of these drugs are currently available in the United Kingdom or have been tested but, at this time, are not indicated for the management of these types of conjunctivitis. In the 1970's and early 1980's, therapeutic approaches to seasonal conjunctivitis were dominated by the use of sodium cromoglycate and with the use of ocular corticosteroids as the next step (see below).

The non-steroidal anti-inflammatory drugs (NSAID's) currently available as ophthalmic products in the UK are diclofenac [*dye-cloe-fen-ac*] sodium 0.1 % (PoM **Voltarol**[R] **Ophtha**) and ketorolac [*key-toe-row-lac*] tromethamine 0.5 % (PoM **Acular**[R]); these eye drops are however <u>not</u> indicated for management of cases of non-infectious, inflammatory conjunctivitis in the UK (although are indicated for this purpose in North America); their use in the UK is as a pre- and post-operative drug for management of inflammation in cataract surgery. However, while their efficacy in acute-onset, short-term therapy or chronic therapy of non-infectious conjunctivitis has not been well established, they are available for this use in North America as an alternative to mild corticosteroid therapy especially in chronic cases, wherefore these eye drops are recommended for use on a *q.d.s.* basis. Supplemental therapy with topical anti-histamines (e.g. naphazoline - antazoline combinations) will probably be required to reduce residual itching, etc. They should not normally be needed for more than 4 to 6 weeks before oedema has resolved and the eye can be managed with mast cell stabilizers, etc.

An ophthalmic NSAID ointment was marketed in the UK for many years but discontinued in 1992. This oxyphenbutazone (PoM **Tanderil**[R]), as a 10 % ointment, was indicated for use as a general anti-inflammatory drug for conditions affecting the conjunctiva and cornea. Over a 40 year period of use in Europe and the UK, it was tried on a wide spectrum of conditions including management of contact lens-related abrasions of the cornea. It is still listed in the formulary for optometrists.

6. MILD OPHTHALMIC CORTICOSTEROID PREPARATIONS

Concurrent use of ophthalmic corticosteroids in non-infectious conjunctivitis is an important option to manage chronic non-infectious inflammation of the conjunctiva. While ophthalmic NSAID's have been introduced in North America and Europe for severe allergic conjunctivitis and related conditions (as "steroid sparing" therapies), in the UK these cases may need to be managed with the periodic or concurrent use of ophthalmic corticosteroids. Topical ocular corticosteroid use is an option for management of chronic and severe cases of conjunctivitis and dilute solutions of clobetasone (e.g 0.1 % as PoM **Cloburate**[R]) or fluorometholone (0.1 % as PoM **FML**[R]) can be used on a chronic basis providing adverse reactions do not develop. For these types of conditions, the dosing for the corticosteroids should be *t.d.s*. If possible, the treatment strategy should be a periodic one, i.e. the steroid eye drops should <u>only</u> be used when the condition is severe, should be used for 1 to 2 weeks and then should be *tapered* (see chapter 13) and eventually discontinued.

When used concurrently with other eye drops, the corticosteroid eye drops should be instilled 15 to 30 minutes after the use of decongestants or mast cell stabilisers since these will help reduce lacrimation and thus improve corticosteroid delivery to the conjunctiva. For some patients, an alternative day steroid use (*q.o.d*) may be sufficient to control symptoms and keep inflammation to a minimum. With either approach, patient follow-up is important to evaluate efficacy, compliance, as to check for possible side effects of steroid therapy.

7. ORAL ANTI-HISTAMINES for CONJUNCTIVITIS.

For cases where ocular symptoms are accompanied by systemic symptoms (e.g. watery eyes accompanied by nasal congestion or a "runny nose"), the use of <u>certain</u> oral histamine H_1 blockers (oral anti-histamines) can be very beneficial. In more severe but predictable chronic cases of allergic conjunctivitis (or rhino-conjunctivitis), systemic administration of these anti-histamines is generally indicated. The easiest way to do this is to instruct on the use of Pharmacy Medicines, although are now available as GSL products.

(**S/P**) Since these anti-histamines have some sympathomimetic potential, their use in patients with known cardiac disease, significant blood pressure disorders or any disorder that might predispose them to cardiac arrhythmias is not recommended. Concurrent administration of other drugs with sympathomimetic potential (MAO inhibitors, NARI's, etc.) should be done cautiously. None of these oral anti-histamine drugs are generally recommended for children, but can be administered at half the adult dosing.

(C/I) (INT) A general warning for an adverse drug reaction (ADR) was issued in 1994 for use of some of these products (especially terfenadine); this warning is now a contra-indication for the use of terfenadine in that it should not be taken concurrently with oral erythromycin, ketoconazole or itraconazole; processed grapefruit juice should also be avoided. These anti-infective drugs and the processed grapefruit juice can substantially reduce the rate of biotransformation and thus the bioelimination of the anti-histamines. As a result, the patient gets an "overdose" with even standard dosing. At high doses, these anti-histamines can precipitate severe cardiac arrhythmias and were fatal in a very few cases.

(i) chlorpheniramine [*klor-fen-eer-a'-meen*] (e.g. P **Piriton**^{R} or P **Calimal**^{R}). Available in blister packs of 30 tablets each containing 4 mg. Numerous generic products containing 4 mg chlorpheniramine are also available. Dosing can be up to *q* 4 h, i.e. up to *q.d.s.*

(ii) acrivastine [*a'cri-va'steen*] (e.g. P **Benadryl Allergy Relief**^{R}). Available in blister packs of 12 or 24 tablets. Dosing may be up to *q* 6 h.

(iii) clemastine [*klem-a'-steen*] (e.g. P/ SL **Aller-Eze**^{R}, P **Tavegil**^{R}). Available in blister packs of 10, 30 or 60 tablets each containing 1 mg. Dosing may be just *b.d.* but can be used up to *q* 4 h.

(iv) loratidine [*lor-a-ti'deen*] (e.g. P **Clarityn**^{R}). Available in blister pack of 7 tablets each containing 10 mg. Once-a-day dosing.

(v) cetirizine [*set-eer-ee-zeen*] (e.g. P/SL **Zirtek**^{R}). Available in blister packs of 7 x 10 mg tablets with a relative cost that is usually 10 X that of chlorpheniramine products for example. Once-a-day dosing.

NOTE. Astemizole [*ah-stem-ee-zole*] was available as an oral anti-histamine as P medicine (e.g. P **Hismanal**^{R}, or P **Pollon-Eze**^{R}) but was switched back to PoM status in mid-1998. The recommended dose was 10 mg *o.d.* (single dose). Terfenadine [*ter-fen-a'deen*], was available as an oral anti-histamine as P Medicine, but reverted to PoM status in September, 1997, and was available in two strengths depending on whether the dosing is *b.d.s.* with 60 mg (PoM **Triludan**^{R}), PoM **Aller-Eze Clear**^{R}) or once-a-day (*o.d.*) with 120 mg (e.g. PoM **Seldane**^{R}, or PoM **Triludan**^{R} **Forte**). Virtually all of these products have now been discontinued. A new terfenadine derivative, fexofenadine (PoM **Telfast**^{R}; now marketed in Australia and Canada OTC) was introduced in 1997and presented as being free from the drug-drug interactions associated with terfenadine (although some ADR's of the type that resulted in the withdrawal of terfenadine and astemizole have been reported). The efficacy of fexofenadine in allergic conjunctivitis remains to be well established.

OPHTHALMIC CORTICOSTEROID PRODUCTS and their USE.

Purpose of chapter. Inflammation of tissues is initiated by vasodilation and release of histamine, prostaglandins and other substances. Such inflammatory responses can be managed, in their early stages, by anti-histamines and non-steroidal anti-inflammatory drugs (NSAID's). However, in more substantial cases of inflammation, stronger anti-inflammatory drugs are needed such as the corticosteroids. The mechanisms of action of these drugs, the reasons for their use and how they should be used are covered in this chapter - to provide an understanding of the use of these drugs by general medical practitioners, as well as ophthalmologists.

MECHANISMS OF CORTICOSTEROIDS and their POTENCY

Corticosteroids can act as *anti-inflammatory* agents, as well as having a number of other effects in the body. Corticosteroids (especially hydrocortisone, also known as cortisol) are normally present in the circulation bind to specific receptors in cells throughout the body. Most corticosteroids used as therapeutics drugs are synthetic but mimic the action of hydrocortisone. The receptors for corticosteroids are unusual in that they are located inside the cells. The activation of these receptors indirectly results in the induced synthesis and release of several peptide hormones and enzymes. One of these peptides is lipocortin-1 which can act as an anti-inflammatory agent by blocking the initial steps in the synthesis of another group of chemicals that cause the tissue inflammatory response; these include arachidonic acid. This initial step of arachidonic acid production requires the activity of an enzyme called phospholipase A_2, which can be inhibited by the lipocortin and as a result, the continued tissue stress does not result in the release of arachidonic acid. This lipocortin inhibition is one step in the production of a range of pro-inflammatory agents since arachidonic acid is also usually biotransformed into a range of compounds called prostaglandins. For this second biotransformation, an enzyme called prostaglandin synthetase is involved and some evidence also suggested that corticosteroids may also suppress synthesis and release of this enzyme.

The corticosteroid anti-inflammatory effect is linked to that of the non-steroidal anti-inflammatory drugs. The NSAID's act to inhibit one of the enzymes involved in the biotransformation of arachidonic acid to prostaglandins; this enzyme is generally referred to as prostaglandin synthetase and is inhibited by a number of NSAID's.

The administration of (synthetic) corticosteroids is essential to control severe inflammation. Minor and moderate reactions of the innate or specific immune system can often be managed by use of drugs that are indirectly active against the vasodilators that promote and sustain the inflammatory response, i.e. vasoconstrictors and NSAID's. When the reaction is more substantial, corticosteroid anti- inflammatory drugs are needed. These corticosteroids serve to directly attenuate the local tissue reactions (including vasodilation, oedema, pain etc.). IF administered early enough, such corticosteroid use should prevent disruptions of the vascular system (that would lead to significant tissue infiltration by white blood cells).

There are a wide range of corticosteroids which are used systemically. Hydrocortisone [*hye-droe-cor-ti-sone*] is used orally (e.g. PoM **Hydrocortistab**[R]) or topically, with the topical (skin) preparations being available as Pharmacy Medicines (e.g. P **HC-45**[R]). Corticosteroids such as beclomethasone [*beck-loh-meth-ah-sone*] are widely used as topical preparations or sprays (e.g. beclomethasone nasal spray; P **Beconase Hayfever**[R]). Triamcinolone [*try-am-sin-oh-lone*] is also used in topical preparations (including those for the ear, e.g. PoM **Tri-Adcortyl**[R] **Otic**) as stronger alternatives to hydrocortisone, but can be taken orally or injected as well. Prednisone and prednisolone [*pred-niss-sol-one*; e.g. PoM **Deltacortril**[R]) are used orally, in topical preparations and by injection (*i.m.*), especially for arthritis conditions and are considered moderate-to-potent steroids. Drugs such as diflucortolone [*dye-flu-cort-oh-lone*] are very potent steroids and generally used in topical preparations (PoM **Nerisone**[R]).

Corticosteroids take a relatively long time to act (i.e. on a time scale of days, rather than hours or minutes) because their receptors are intracellular and the mechanism indirect. Equally importantly, a long time period is also required for the effects of corticosteroid therapy to cease after the administration of these drugs has been stopped. Therefore, for clinically useful effects to occur, corticosteroids might need to be given for several days before any effect is really apparent; this represents a difficult therapeutic strategy. When corticosteroids are used, especially systemically, there is always a chance that the natural immune system can be suppressed as well. Corticosteroids are sometimes deliberately used in very high doses as immunosuppressants (to prevent tissue rejection or other severe reactions). However, their long term use at normal doses always carries a risk of unwanted suppression of the body's natural ability to fight infection.

CORTICOSTEROIDS for OPHTHALMIC USE

Ophthalmic corticosteroid preparations are indicated for use whenever there is inflammation present, or a risk of this developing. Plasma levels of hydrocortisone can show a marked diurnal variation and the vascular system of the eye (including the secretion of the aqueous humour, and thus IOP) is probably regulated by these cyclical changes. The development of tissue oedema (including in the eye) will thus depend upon natural corticosteroid levels, and the addition of corticosteroids as medications is thus a supplement to a natural mechanism and regulatory cycle. The corticosteroids also serve to directly reduce leakiness of the vasculature of the anterior uvea and reduce the rate of migration of white blood cells into the ocular tissues.

Topical ophthalmic corticosteroids are available as eye drops or ointments, and often in combination with anti-infective drugs (chapter 16). Ocular corticosteroids are sometimes referred to as a palliative (or cover up) therapy. However, since corticosteroids achieve their anti-inflammatory effects by increasing release of inflammation-blocking mediators such as lipocortin-1, and reducing the release of cyclooxygenase enzymes such as COX-2 that produce inflammatory mediators such as prostaglandins), they do generally counteract the inflammatory process. Some however might argue that the overall action of corticosteroids is indirect, and that they do nothing to "directly" counter the cause of the inflammation. From the latter perspective, the corticosteroids merely act - after the fact - to attenuate the inflammatory response. With our current understanding of the molecular mechanisms of corticosteroid action, it seems more appropriate to not only specifically designate corticosteroids as being indirect-acting drugs, but also that they are a "cure" for the inflammation, and not simply a cover-up. Regardless of one's perspective, the palliative designation does have an important clinical consequence in that all ophthalmic corticosteroids should only be carefully used under supervision. When used in this way, they are extraordinarily effective and safe therapeutic drugs.

A.   General Indications for use of ophthalmic corticosteroids.

There are many indications for local therapy of the eye with corticosteroids and these can also be supplemented with systemic (oral) corticosteroids in severe cases. There are many uses of ophthalmic corticosteroids in cases of inflammation associated with infections but their primary use is for non-infectious inflammatory disorders -

(**a**) associated with chronic chemical or drug irritation of the eyelids that leads to oedema of the eyelid margins and palpebral conjunctiva, e.g. those associated with severe allergic reactions of any type, severe seasonal allergies, acute or sub-acute allergic blepharitis from airborne sources or contact with chemicals or drugs, severe inflammation associated with chemical contact (alkali burns), or select cases of lid gland dysfunction.

(**b**) chronic irritation of the palpebral or bulbar conjunctiva associated with repeated exposure to allergens, or chemical vapors (e.g. vernal conjunctivitis), or associated with mechanical - chemical irritation (e.g. giant papillary conjunctivitis following contact lens wear).

(**c**) for superficial punctate keratitis (SPK) of almost any etiology, generalized diffuse keratitis of a non-infectious etiology, chemical (toxic) keratitis and where there is non-ulcerating active stromal involvement.

(**d**) for acute, sub-acute or chronic inflammatory conditions of the sclera, anterior uveal tract, iris and cornea associated with mechanical (including any surgical or para-surgical procedure), chemical or bacterial trauma.

(**e**) for adjunct use in generalised <u>iritis and anterior uveitis</u> associated with systemic disorders (e.g. arthritis) and select acute or sub-acute cases of episcleritis or scleritis. These disorders generally also require systemic steroid use because of their recurrent or chronic nature.

B. <u>Ophthalmic corticosteroid-containing products</u>.

Ophthalmic corticosteroids and the different products can be ranked approximately in order of increasing anti-inflammatory action. This is very important because, as with the systemic use of corticosteroids, ophthalmic corticosteroid selection is largely done on the expected drug potency rather than its concentration or dosing regimen. For mild-to-moderate inflammations, mild-to-moderate potency corticosteroids are indicated for periodic use; for severe inflammations, moderate-to-strong corticosteroids are indicated for periodic or intensive use. All ophthalmic corticosteroid preparations in the UK are Prescription-only Medicines, and most are preserved with benzalkonium chloride.

(**i**) hydrocortisone. This steroid, as its acetate derivative, has a relative ophthalmic anti-inflammatory activity of 1. This ophthalmic corticosteroid was introduced in the 1950's and is not widely used nowadays. Hydrocortisone, as eye drops or the ointment form, can be used for relatively superficial non-infectious inflammatory conditions of the lids or conjunctiva where there is no major defect or signs of ulceration. Numerous hydrocortisone products are marketed at the 1 % strength as an ophthalmic suspension (eye drops, PoM **Hydrocortisone**, generic, 10 mL bottle). There is also hydrocortisone 0.5 %, 1 % and 2.5 % in ointment form (PoM **Hydrocortisone**, generic, 3 g tubes). These will be used by hospitals because they are so cheap. A number of combination products with anti-bacterial drugs are also marketed (see chapter 16).

(**ii**) clobetasone. This steroid, as its butyrate derivative, has a relative ophthalmic anti-inflammatory activity of 2. It is generally indicated for milder inflammatory conditions. It is available at the 0.1 % concentration in eye drops (e.g. PoM **Cloburate**[R], 10 mL bottles). No generics listed.

(**iii**) betamethasone. This steroid, as its sodium phosphate salt has an ophthalmic anti-inflammatory activity of 3 to 4. It is thus indicated for use in moderate inflammatory conditions. of the lids, conjunctiva, cornea and anterior segment associated with allergic, chemical or mechanical trauma. It is available at the 0.1 % concentration as eye drops (e.g. PoM **Betnesol**[R], 10 mL bottle, and PoM **Vista-Methasone**[R], 5 mL and 10 mL bottles) and also in an ophthalmic ointment at the 0.1 % concentration (PoM **Betnesol**[R], 3 g tube). No generics listed. Some combination products with antibiotics are also marketed. It is widely used by GP's and ophthalmologists probably because it is cheap (especially the ointment).

(**iv**) dexamethasone. This steroid, as its sodium phosphate or sodium metasulphobenzoate derivatives, has a relative ophthalmic anti-inflammatory activity of 4. It is generally indicated for use in moderate inflammations but can be used intensively for severe inflammations (including as a post-operative corticosteroid). Available as eye drops at the 0.1 % concentration with hypromellose 0.5 % in 5 mL or 10 mL bottles as (e.g. PoM **Maxidex**^{R}) and as **Minims**^{R} **Dexamethasone**, unit-dose. No generic products are currently listed. Some combinations with anti-bacterial drugs are available.

(**v**) prednisolone. This is probably the most widely used ophthalmic corticosteroid because it is available at two concentrations as different derivatives to cover a wide spectrum of diseases.The sodium phosphate derivatives are generally considered to have a relative ophthalmic anti-inflammatory activity of 3 or 5 (depending on the strength used) and are indicated for use in moderate inflammations. The acetate derivative is considered by some to have slightly superior anti-inflammatory activity and thus indicated for moderate or severe inflammations. Prednisolone sodium phosphate ophthalmic solution (eye drops) is available at the 0.5 % concentration (e.g. PoM **Predsol**^{R}, 10 mL bottle, **Minims**^{R} **Prednisolone**, unit-dose), prednisolone acetate ophthalmic suspension (eye drops) is available at the 1 % concentration (e.g. PoM **Pred Forte**^{R}, 5 mL and 10 mL bottles). No generic products, but a number of combination products with anti-bacterial drugs are marketed.

(**vi**) fluorometholone. This steroid, as its base, has an ophthalmic anti-inflammatory activity of 5 but is used (in the UK) at a low concentration (i.e. 0.1 %) so is generally indicated for mild-to-moderate inflammations when a rapid response is deemed appropriate. Fluorometholone is available as eye drops at 0.1 % concentration with polyvinyl alcohol (PoM **FML**^{R} Liquifilm, 5 mL or 10 mL bottles). Combination products with anti-bacterial drugs are also available.

(**vii**) a new ophthalmic corticosteroid, rimexolone, was introduced in the USA in late 1995 (VEXOL™) primarily of post-surgical use similar to **Pred Forte**^{R}. This is the first of a group of 'soft' corticosteroids that have substantial anti-inflammatory effects (probably equivalent to prednisolone 1 %) but are biotransformed so rapidly to what appear to be largely inactive metabolites that the side effects profile is lessened. Long term clinical experience has yet to be reported with this type of drug. Another soft ophthalmic corticosteroid, loteprednol, was marketed in the USA in 1998 (as both APREX™ and LOTEMAX™). Its use is primary as a post-operative corticosteroid but can also be used for general non-infected inflammatory conditions of the conjunctiva and cornea.

NOTE. In the 1970's and into the 1980's, another ophthalmic corticosteroid was widely used. Medrysone (HMS LIQUIFILM^R), as a 1 % ophthalmic suspension, has a relative activity of 2. It was indicated for use in mild chronic inflammatory conditions of the conjunctiva (e.g. seasonal or vernal conjunctivitis) where steroid therapy was thought desirable.

C. Clinical efficacy of ophthalmic corticosteroids and their use.

(**a**) dosing for topical ocular corticosteroids therapy should be started at q 4 h or q 6 h, when the presenting signs are mild to moderate. The corticosteroid product is selected based on relative activity (see above). In really severe cases, especially following surgery or acute-onset iritis or anterior uveitis, ophthalmic corticosteroids (especially dexamethasone or prednisolone) may be used q 2 h, usually for the first 24 h only. In most cases, ophthalmic corticosteroid preparations are for short-term use only and this time period appears to be designated as 3 weeks maximum. Treatment of moderate-to-severe inflammation with topical ocular corticosteroids should result in some improvement (in both symptoms and signs) within 48 h and a definite improvement within 7 days; if this does not occur, the corticosteroid therapy should be reconsidered (see later). However, when used to correct chronic inflammation of the lids or conjunctiva, it may take many days to a couple of weeks before a definite improvement is observed. Thus, in some cases, a decision will need to be made as to whether the condition continues to be managed at the primary care level (including by a general medical practitioner) or should be referred to an ophthalmologist.

(**b**) follow-up after starting ocular corticosteroid therapy. Periodic examinations (circa q. 2 weeks) are necessary to monitor the efficacy of the steroid regimen and allow appropriate changes in regimen. Ocular corticosteroid use should not be embarked upon without ensuring that routine and regular follow-up is possible, especially if longer term treatment is anticipated (i.e. over 3 weeks). For acute conditions and depending on the severity of the condition, these checks are generally made at 3 and 7 days and then every 4 to 7 days thereafter until substantial resolution of the condition has occurred (as evidenced by diminution of symptoms and clear reduction of the signs of inflammation). The ocular assessment should cover general inspection (including eyelid eversion and inspection), biomicroscopy (including evaluation of the anterior chamber for any reaction / flare / cells etc.) and evaluation of the pupil / iris (especially for signs of acute inflammatory reaction). Patient records should include notes as to the magnitude of the oedema and should be made such that some degree of objectivity is possible in deciding the degree of resolution, or otherwise of any corneal oedema and other reactions at both central and more peripheral sites. The follow-up is also necessary so that the following can be (re)considered -

(i) (S/P) <u>concurrent bacterial infections</u>. Corticosteroid therapy of the eye is contraindicated in purulent infections. Corticosteroid therapy, while an essential part of management of tissue inflammation, can interfere with and mask concurrent bacterial infections; any indication that the inflammation is getting worse (including appearance of extra discharge and mucus) should prompt consideration of whether there is an underlying infection. Any infectious condition should be managed promptly (see chapters 15 and 16). The eye-quietening effects of successful corticosteroid therapy means that the eye may not show all of the expected early signs and symptoms of an infection.

(ii) (C/I) <u>concurrent active HSV infection</u>. Ocular corticosteroid therapy is contraindicated in the presence of an active viral infection. The reason for the contraindication applies primarily to herpes simplex (HSV) infections. Inflamed eyes will generally be painful and patient presents with moderate-to-profuse lacrimation (especially in acute phases) but these could equally well be indicative of an HSV infection; concurrent corticosteroid use can exacerbate an active HSV keratitis. While part of the initial evaluation (including fluorescein use and biomicroscopy) should be to rule out HSV as a cause of the problems, the use of stains and biomicroscopy should be done at check-up visits for the presence of even the smallest corneal surface lesion. Some also recommend that other viral infections should also not be managed initially with corticosteroids.

(iii) (C/I) <u>concurrent fungal or protozoan infections</u>.Ophthalmic corticosteroid therapy is contraindicated in the presence of active fungal or protozoan infections. Concurrent steroid use may exacerbate an active fungal or protozoan infection of the eye. *Acanthamoeba* infections in contact lens-wearers is the current concern but any history that includes certain risk factors for protozoan or fungal infections (e.g. known vegetative injury to the eye, hot tub use, use of homemade saline solutions with contact lens wear) should be taken as sufficient circumstantial evidence to require that cultures are taken (see chapters 16 and 17), and to keep corticosteroid therapy to a minimum until further diagnosis is made.

(iv) (C/I) <u>active tuberculosis infections</u>. Ophthalmic corticosteroid therapy is contraindicated when there is an *active* tubercle infection (Tb). Concurrent corticosteroid use could exacerbate any tubercle-related disease of the conjunctiva as well as the rest of the eye. Any patient with ocular inflammation and a history of Tb infections requires a comprehensive work up, which should include evaluation of the status of their past Tb-related problems (and re-instigation of, or changing of medications for Tb).

(v) <u>IOP</u>. Listings for ophthalmic corticosteroids in the MIMS and BNF include a warning (caution) about the possibility of an adverse drug reaction (**ADR**); this may be referred to as "steroid glaucoma" or raised intra-ocular pressure. Corticosteroid eye drop use can increase IOP to unacceptable levels and this needs to be checked for at each patient assessment. A small percentage of the population (exact number etc., uncertain) display an unusual ocular response to topical ocular corticosteroids in that, over a period of 2 to 3 weeks, their IOP increases to over 30 mm Hg (and can increase much further if corticosteroid therapy is not reduced). The older corticosteroids (e.g. hydrocortisone) and those indicated for and used aggressively to manage moderate-to-severe inflammations (e.g. dexamethasone or prednisolone) may increase IOP's more than other corticosteroids (e.g. clobetasone or fluorometholone). This potential difference in ADR does <u>not</u> however mean that patients prescribed clobetasone or fluorometholone eye drops do not need to be monitored regularly. The patients that develop an increased IOP are thought to have a genetic predisposition to such corticosteroid-induced ocular hypertension; these patients are known as "steroid responders". The IOP however should return to normal levels over 1 to 2 weeks when corticosteroid therapy is tapered and discontinued. Therefore, IOP must be monitored periodically, especially in longer-term therapy to identify these responders; "periodically" can be translated to every 10 to 14 days. The ADR warning is such that some recommend that ophthalmic corticosteroid therapies of longer than 3 weeks should only be carried out under the supervision of an ophthalmologist.

(vi) (S/P) <u>re-epithelialization, ocular surface re-healing and corneal thinning</u>. Excessive topical ocular corticosteroid therapy *may* retard the natural re-surfacing / healing processes of the surface membranes. Corticosteroid therapies should thus be limited to q 4 or q 6 h (except in initial management of severe and acute-onset conditions). Such retarded wound healing may result in further oedema developing (because the barrier function of the epithelium is not re-established) as well as predispose the ocular surface to recurrent or secondary infection. Similarly, indiscriminate and unsupervised use of ophthalmic corticosteroids can produce progressive thinning of the corneal stroma, especially in the periphery.

(vii) (S/P) <u>ending corticosteroid therapy</u>. Wherever possible, ocular corticosteroid therapy should not be abruptly discontinued. The palliative effects of corticosteroid therapy mean that the usual indicators of inflammation will be lessened. Slowly reducing corticosteroid therapy should allow one to see how inflamed the eye still is and avoid there being an acute rebound response of the eye without corticosteroid anti-inflammatory therapy. This <u>tapering</u> of corticosteroid therapy (e.g. from ongoing therapy at q 4 h to q 6 h, reduce to *b.d.* and then to *o.d.* after a day or so) allows adequate evaluation of the extent of any associated-infection and the true status of the corneal and conjunctival surfaces.

OPHTHALMIC ANTI-BACTERIAL DRUGS and their USES

Purpose of chapter. Bacterial infections of the external eye should be promptly evaluated and treated. Current scope of optometric practice includes the "emergency" management of such conditions. In this chapter, the properties of the currently-marketed ophthalmic anti-bacterial drugs will be outlined, and details are provided on how they should be used.

Different pharmaceuticals are available to manage the different types of bacterial infection that can affect the lids, conjunctiva and cornea, providing that the organisms are sensitive to the anti-bacterial drugs being used. In considering the use and selection of these products, several things need to be considered. Diagnosis / recognition of an infection (or condition at risk for developing an infection), selection of the appropriate primary and secondary therapeutic measures, instigating treatment and / or providing treatment, or prescribing anti-bacterial drugs and consideration of the availability of follow-up are all important.

Knowledge of current availability of ophthalmic anti-bacterial drugs is important, so that appropriate decisions can be made on each of these issues. Ophthalmic anti-bacterials fall into different categories which generally reflect the severity of the infection that needs to be treated.

1. *General purpose, BROAD SPECTRUM antibiotics*. These are suitable for management of acute onset, moderate-to-severe bacterial infections of the external eye. Their usage is often very selective and based upon practitioner preference; some of these drugs have thus become far more widely used than others. Such preferences for drug type or product should <u>not</u> be taken as true measures of efficacy since, regardless of how popular a product or drug is, efficacy can only be based on observing that a bacterial infection is rapidly eliminated. This is determined by the bacterial susceptibility to the drugs, <u>and</u> patient compliance with the recommended treatment regimen. Overall however, all of the broad spectrum anti-bacterial drugs (products) can be expected to show similar efficacy when used appropriately to manage infections that have resulted from the presence of susceptible gram-negative or gram-positive bacteria. The selection of products will be, in part, determined by choices of anti-bacterial / corticosteroid products (see chapter 16), and by experience on which products are found to be adequate to manage infections, especially unresponsive ones.

(**a**) chloramphenicol. This broad spectrum antibiotic is an inhibitor of protein synthesis in bacteria. It has been used to great positive effect in ophthalmic products for very many years, since its introduction in the 1950's. Chloramphenicol ophthalmic products are widely used by general medical practitioners, as well as other health care practitioners. It can be used and supplied by optometrists on an "emergency" basis, and is indicated for use to manage bacterial infections of the lids, conjunctiva and cornea. It is widely available as 0.5 % eye drops (e.g. PoM **Minims**^R **Chloramphenicol** eye drops, unit dose; PoM **Chloromycetin**^R Redidrops, 5 mL or 10 mL bottles; PoM **Sno Phenicol**^R, 10 mL bottles); numerous generic products containing chloramphenicol 0.5 % for ophthalmic use are also available and all are inexpensive. Chloramphenicol eye drops need to be refrigerated. Ointments containing 1 % chloramphenicol are also available (e.g. PoM **Chloromycetin**^R, PoM **Chloramphenicol Eye Ointment**, both 4 g tubes) with a number of other generic ointment products usually marketed as well. A combination product with corticosteroids is also available (see chapter 16).

(**S/P**) Chloramphenicol ophthalmic products are not intended for chronic use, nor even repeated regularly for short-term therapies. (**C/I**) / (**ADR**) A small note in the directory listings for ophthalmic chloramphenicol states that an Adverse Drug Reaction is aplastic anaemia; this note also states that this reaction is rare, and current epidemiological studies clearly support this perspective. It is not really possible to identify who might be at risk for developing such a potentially-fatal adverse reaction which probably arises because of a pharmacogenetic difference in metabolism of this drug. Such a note, or its equivalent, has been on some chloramphenicol products for over 20 years.A few medical practitioners have expressed concern that a use of chloramphenicol eye drops constitutes an unacceptable (and avoidable) risk. Such concerns once prompted some hospitals to state that chloramphenicol should only be used when other ophthalmic antibiotics have failed to produce the desired effects.

Any optometrist in the UK can initiate treatment with chloramphenicol eye drops or ointment, and supply an appropriate quantity of the pharmaceuticals to a patient for self-administration (see Chapter 19). Within such an "emergency" perspective, the optometrist should be prepared to be completely responsible for the well-being of the patient under treatment, including appropriate follow-up care and check-ups.

(**b**) framycetin. This is an aminoglycoside antibiotic related to neomycin. Framycetin, as an aminoglycoside, inhibits protein synthesis in bacteria but by a different mechanism to chloramphenicol. It is indicated for use in the management of styes, blepharitis and bacterial conjunctivitis, corneal abrasions and even burns and peripheral ulcers. Framycetin is available at the 0.5 % concentration in eye drops (**Soframycin**^R, 10 mL bottle) as in ointment form (PoM **Soframycin**^R, 5 g tube; inexpensive). It is indicated for use in the management of styes, blepharitis and bacterial conjunctivitis, corneal abrasions and even burns and ulcers. The drug is listed on the optometry formulary, so can theoretically be used by optometrists on an "emergency" basis (see Chapter 19). (**S/P**) Patients may show cross-reactivity with other aminoglycosides such as neomycin and gentamicin. A product with corticosteroids is also available (see chapter 16).

(**c**) gentamicin. This is another aminoglycoside antibiotic (protein synthesis inhibitor) and a common choice for a prescription-only broad spectrum anti-bacterial eye drops. It is indicated for use in any bacterial infections of the cornea and conjunctiva, including severe infections and ulcers susceptible to gentamicin. It is not currently approved for general use by optometrists. It is available at the 0.3 % concentration in eye drops (e.g. PoM **Minims**[R] **Gentamicin**, unit dose; PoM **Cidomycin**[R] Eyedrops, 8 mL bottle; PoM **Garamycin**[R] Eyedrops, 10 mL bottle; and PoM **Genticin**[R] Eyedrops, 10 mL bottle). An ophthalmic ointment of gentamicin 0.3 % was discontinued in late 1998 (PoM **Cidomycin Eye Ointment**[R], 5 g tube) (**S/P**) Gentamicin ophthalmic products may elicit local allergic or otherwise irritating reactions in patients sensitive to this or other aminoglycoside antibiotics (e.g. neomycin and framycetin).

(**d**) neomycin. This is broad spectrum aminoglycoside (protein synthesis inhibitor) antibiotic, that was once widely used on its own for bacterial infections of the eye. It is indicated for use in the management of styes, blepharitis and bacterial conjunctivitis, corneal abrasions and keratitis. It is not currently approved for general use by optometrists. It is now only marketed on its own in brand products as PoM **Minims**[R] **Neomycin** Eyedrops (unit dose), although generic products of both the eye drops (3500 units/mL) and ophthalmic ointment (3500 units/g) are also available (PoM **Neomycin**, generic). Combination products with other antibiotics are available (see below) as are a number of specific combination products with ophthalmic corticosteroids (see chapter 16). (**S/P**) Allergies; neomycin is considered, by some, to be the aminoglycoside that is most likely to precipitate allergic reactions of the lids and peri-ocular skin. If such an ADR develops, therapy should be discontinued.

(**e**) fusidic acid (also known as fusidate sodium) (PoM **Fucithalmic**[R], 5 g tube). This is another protein synthesis inhibitor but which has a slightly narrower spectrum than related drugs, although overall can be expected to have a similar efficacy to chloramphenicol and gentamicin when susceptible organisms are the cause of bacterial infections of the conjunctiva. It is not meant for use in severe infections. It is not currently approved for general use by optometrists. It is available as a unique viscous eye drop at the 1 % concentration, for *b.d.s.* usage, that can be especially useful for children. The viscous preparation is applied as if it were an ointment, but which then readily mixes with the tear film.

(**f**) fluoroquinolones such as ciprofloxacin 0.3 % ([*si-proe-flox-a'sin*]; PoM **Ciloxan**[R], 5 mL bottle) and ofloxacin 0.3 % ([*oh'flox-a'sin*]; PoM **Exocin**[R], 5 mL bottle). These anti-bacterial drugs have similar broad-spectrum efficacy to gentamicin, but work by an entirely different mechanism by blocking DNA synthesis in bacteria. The fluoroquinolones are currently primarily indicated for the management of corneal ulcers, although they should also be effective in combatting a wide range of bacterial infections of the external eye (including conjunctivitis). They are not currently approved for use by optometrists. Ointment formulations with ciprofloxacin are now marketed in Canada, and ointments containing ofloxacin are currently being tested in clinical trials. The fluoroquinolones have proved to be useful alternatives to aminoglycosides, when aminoglycoside-resistant bacterial strains have been encountered but, in their own right, some unexpected resistance development has been noted as well. (ADR) Conjunctival concretions (small diffuse punctate deposits of crystallized drugs) can be an annoying side effect. The suitability of fluoroquinolone use in children has yet to be fully defined.

NOTE. Another aminoglycoside antibiotic, tobramycin was available until 1997, when manufacture for UK distribution (as PoM **Tobralex**[R] 0.3 %) was discontinued. It was often used as the first alternative to gentamicin or as a first choice drug by some practitioners, with an efficacy and spectrum of activity similar to gentamicin. The product may still be specially imported for hospital clinic use for severe susceptible infections.

2. *general purpose ophthalmic anti-bacterials*. These drugs are principally for mild-to-moderate infections of the conjunctiva and eyelids. These drugs (or drug combinations) are used for minor external eye and eyelid infections (including many childhood infections), and for prophylaxis against similar infections. In many of these types of cases there is simply no need for use of a high efficacy, potent broad-spectrum anti-bacterial drug. Adequate management can be achieved with the use of these often-cheaper anti-infectives when used frequently at high doses, or when used as mixtures of several anti-bacterial drugs at low concentrations. Such products are not meant for use in severe bacterial infection, especially when the condition is associated with substantial mucopurulent discharge and inflammation.

These general purpose products use an alternative approach to a broad-spectrum profile in that two or more anti-bacterial drugs are included in one pharmaceutical; both gram-positive and gram-negative organisms should be acted upon. Bacitracin provides coverage against gram-positive organisms, while polymyxin B and gramicidin are the drugs that provide coverage against gram-negative organisms. These products are not currently approved for general use by optometrists.

Examples of general purpose anti-bacterial drugs include combinations of polymyxin B with bacitracin as PoM **Polyfax**[R], 4 g tubes), trimethoprim (a sulpha-type drug; see below) and polymyxin B (as PoM **Polytrim**[R], 5 mL bottles; as ointment in PoM **Polytrim**[R] Ointment, 4 g tubes), and combinations of polymyxin B, gramicidin and neomycin (as PoM **Neosporin**[R], 5 mL bottles; expensive !).

Other general purpose anti-bacterial drugs include propamidine isethionate or dibromopropamidine isethionate. These drugs have general antibiotic actions, but - when evaluated in the 1940's - showed excellent efficacy against the common gram positive bacteria that caused cases of conjunctivitis, styes and generalised blepharitis, e.g. *Staphylococcus* sp and many *Streptococcus* sp. Their activity against these organisms is largely unaffected by muco-purulent discharge. Their mechanism of action include blocking purine nucleotide uptake by bacteria, and thus indirectly to block DNA synthesis. These two drugs are available as Pharmacy Medicines as both eye drops (P **Golden Eye**[R], 10 mL bottle; P **Brolene**[R], 10 mL bottle; 0.1 % concentration) or an ophthalmic ointment (P **Golden Eye Ointment**[R] or P **Brolene**[R] Eye ointment; 3.5 g tubes). (**S/P**) A recommendation should be given that (medical) attention should be sought if the condition does not show signs of improvement within 2 days.

NOTE. Sulphonamide drugs. The "sulpha" (sulphonamide) drugs are still to found in the printed version of the optometrists formulary (Chapter 19). The formulary lists sulphacetamide sodium, mafenide and sulphafurazole as being available as prescription-only products for optometric use on an "emergency" basis. These drugs are not currently available in commercial products in the UK for ophthalmic use, although sulphacetamide eye drops could perhaps be prepared by a major hospital pharmacy. The last product (PoM **Albucid**[R] eye drops) was discontinued in 1993. These drugs are generally more effective against gram-positive organisms (that are the commoner causes of uncomplicated bacterial infections of the external eye) but show reduced efficacy if there is substantial muco-purulent discharge. Sulphacetamide was usually used at the 10 % concentration (in eye drops or ointments) but could be used at the 30 % concentration as eye drops. The drug is still widely available in the USA and Canada.

3. OTHER ophthalmic anti-bacterials with select uses.

Fortified antibiotics are for severe, ulcerating infections of the cornea, certain antibiotics can be prepared as special concentrated solutions. In rare cases, an eye does not respond well to either the primary or secondary therapy, continues to deteriorate and is now a severe infection. In such cases it is not only important to manage the bacterial infection with an antibiotic with proven efficacy against the bacterial strain responsible for the infection (and this can only be done providing laboratory culture tests have been performed with isolates obtained from the infected eye) but it is also very important that this antibiotic therapy should now be extraordinarily intensive; this is the use of the "fortified" antibiotic preparations. These preparations can only be made in a hospital pharmacy as and when needed, and will often only be prepared on a daily basis. These preparations are not listed in pharmaceutical directories. Most of these preparations have short shelf lives and are unpreserved. The concentration of the antibiotic may be 2 to 5 times higher than that in commercially-available products. These products will initially be used at *q* 15 to *q* 30 min for 24 h but then may later be used at *q* 1 to *q* 4 h, or a regular antibiotic product used instead after the saturation dosing with the fortified antibiotic. Some of the more commonly used fortified antibiotics are fortified 1 % gentamicin, neomycin, or vancomycin solutions for identified gram-positive infections; fortified polymyxin B solutions may be used for identified gram-negative infections.

USE OF OPHTHALMIC ANTIBACTERIAL PRODUCTS

There are several things to be considered -

1. recognition of an infection as being bacterial in origin as opposed to viral, fungal or protozoan. Bacterial infections of the eyelid margins often leave substantial encrustation on the eyelashes; bacterial infection of the conjunctiva is usually accompanied by white-yellow stringy / gummy muco-purulent discharge (although similar white and stringy discharge can accompany some acute allergic reactions); the extent of the mucopurulent discharge may be sufficient to make the lids stick together, especially overnight. Viral and fungal infections are more commonly accompanied by profuse tearing without discharge or encrustation. The involvement of the conjunctiva may spread to the cornea and / or a focal involvement of the cornea is present (e.g. from an abrasion or contact lens wear trauma, etc.).

2. history tends to be acute. This is perhaps obvious, but important, since the irritation and /or signs (red eye) associated with the infection is usually sufficient to prompt patients' to seek attention. However, some patients may not seek attention when they have minor infections wherein they are already accustomed to a degree of ocular irritation / discomfort / foreign body sensation, and perhaps a history of recurrent minor infections (that can be largely managed by good ocular hygiene). Rarely encountered will be a patient, through resistance to seeking treatment, who allows a condition to become severe before presenting for attention. Notwithstanding, many bacterial infections will be self-limiting and also may resolve on their own without any specific drug treatment (other than good hygiene measures, that include observance of measures to stop re-infection, and prevent cross-contamination to other family members).

Treatment with anti-bacterials is in order whenever an infection is suspected, or there has been a trauma or abrasion that might become infected, simply because of a compromised corneal or conjunctival epithelium (especially in ill or elderly patients). Hygiene measures may often be preferable in children, rather than anti-bacterial drug prophylaxis.

3. Selection of appropriate primary and secondary therapy. There are three aspects to this which are product selection (i.e. deciding which anti-bacterial drug and pharmaceutical type is appropriate for the condition), deciding on the treatment regimen (i.e. the use of anti-bacterial drugs requires a specific regimen to be stipulated) and predicting the outcome of treatment. The outcome obviously depends on whether the chosen therapy was actually effective against the pathogen. Either an antibacterial drug is chosen and used on a patient (i.e. chloramphenicol), or the patient can be managed on a short-term basis with a small supply of chloramphenicol, or that patient is referred for a prescription to be written for the same or another broad-spectrum antibiotic (or combination of anti-bacterial drugs). This broad-spectrum approach is by far the most widely used and is sometimes called the "shotgun" approach. It carries the inherent risk that the therapy will not be successful and the practitioner is left without samples of the microorganisms for culturing. In severe infections, such samples really need to be taken prior to initiation of treatment and then the treatment started on an urgent basis. Almost all mild-to- moderate conjunctival and eyelid infections can be managed with broad spectrum antibiotics without cultures.

4. practical considerations in PRODUCT SELECTION and USE. All ophthalmic anti-bacterial products are not equal. In selecting a particular pharmaceutical, the following should be considered. First and foremost is the issue of allergies; allergic reactions to ophthalmic antibiotics are the commonest reason for adverse reactions developing during therapy and for the therapy being discontinued. Allergies are more likely to be encountered with the aminoglycosides (e.g. neomycin) compared to other antibiotics, although chloramphenicol could elicit a unique systemic sensitisation (especially if inappropriately used). Other issues include considering whether refrigeration for pharmaceuticals is available (since some ophthalmic antibiotics are remarkably effective but need to be refrigerated, e.g. chloramphenicol eye drops), considering how much discharge there is (since some ophthalmic antibacterial drugs may not be effective in infections where there is a lot of muco-purulent discharge, although ocular irrigation prior to application of the eye drops can reduce this problem) and lastly to consider whether overnight anti-bacterial treatment (" coverage") will be necessary. This coverage generally requires the use of ointments, and some anti-bacterial drug products are only available in solution form and do not have a companion ointment product for overnight coverage. It is perhaps easiest to prescribe from the same line of pharmaceuticals.

5. Regimens for suggested use, and patient education.

(**a**) initial regimen. Any therapy for mild-to-moderate bacterial infections should be instigated at q 4 or q 6 h. If the condition is more severe, all broad spectrum ophthalmic antibacterial drugs can be administered q 2 h during the first 24 h. Ophthalmic gels can be used *b.d.s*, i.e. q 6 to 8 h or "morning and night". The pharmaceuticals chosen and the prescribed regimen should always be noted in the patient's file.

(**b**) duration of therapy. A reasonable regimen is 7 to 10 days with check-up (see below) and most infections should respond substantially over this period (providing the organism was sensitive to the drug or drugs used). The check-up ensures that this response is occurring. An alternative strategy is to stipulate that the treatment should be until 2 or 3 days after the eye infection is no longer apparent and the eye is generally comfortable again.

(**c**) <u>overnight coverage</u>. Wherever possible, an ointment should be used *h.s.* in addition to the *q* 4 h drops; IF the infection is severe, the drops need to be used night and day initially.

(**d**) <u>patient instruction</u>. It should never be assumed that a patient knows how to use the drops or ointment containing an anti-infective; time should be taken to educate them on instillation / application, hygiene, storage and disposal of the pharmaceuticals. Reasonable effort should be extended to ensure that the patient understands the importance of compliance, and in uncertain cases it would be best to dispense an ointment.

(**e**) availability of <u>follow-up</u>. Ideally, no patient should be prescribed anti-infective medications without there being the opportunity for follow-up, i.e. it would be better to refer a patient to someone who can provide the follow-up rather than just dispensing tubes of PoM **Chloromycetin**[R] (or similar), and hoping the infection will be "cured". Depending on the severity of the condition, the first follow-up should be at 24 or 48 hr. For moderate infections, a patient can usually be instructed at a second follow-up visit to continue therapy for one more week (or 2 to 3 days after the eye looks quiet again). In such cases where improvement is occurring, the follow-up could be via a telephone call with the intent of arranging a brief final check if considered appropriate.

Obviously, if an eye appears worse on follow-up then appropriate changes in anti-bacterial therapy and referral, at the very least simply for cultures, is very important. In rare cases, it should always be considered that the infection may not even be bacterial in nature, but due to fungi or a virus.

OTHER OCULAR ANTI-INFECTIVES and THEIR USE.

Purpose of chapter. Optometrists are permitted to manage uncomplicated mild-to-moderate bacterial infections of the external eye on an "emergency" basis, but currently need to refer patients for treatment of severe infections or those requiring extended treatment. For bacterial infections, the use of PoM products containing gentamicin or the fluoroquinolones is often indicated for these types of referral cases. However, there are a variety of other infections that are of a chronic nature that require use of other antibacterials, or there are infections due to viral or fungal pathogens. It is the goal of this chapter to discuss the medical management of milder but often chronic bacterial infections of the external eye. In addition, the options that are available to the specialist to manage viral and fungal infections of the eye will be considered. The supplementary use of cycloplegic drugs as therapeutic agents will also be discussed.

MANAGEMENT OF ACUTE INFECTIONS OF THE LIDS

Styes or many other inflammatory infections of the eyelash follicles, glands or accessory lacrimal glands can be readily managed with instruction on ocular hygiene and the use of several ophthalmic antibiotic ointments. If poorly managed, or complicated by poor hygiene and ill health, these simple conditions can develop into chronic ones and can sometimes be very severe indeed (orbital cellulitis).The antibiotics available include -

(**a**) propamidine isethionate or dibromopropamidine isethionate show good efficacy against the common gram positive bacteria that caused cases of styes and generalised blepharitis, e.g. *Staphylococcus* sp and many *Streptococcus* sp. Their activity against these organisms is largely unaffected by muco-purulent discharge. Their mechanism of action include blocking purine nucleotide uptake by bacteria, and thus indirectly to block DNA synthesis. Available as Pharmacy Medicines as an ophthalmic ointment (P **Golden Eye Ointment**[R] or P **Brolene**[R] Eye ointment; 3.5 g tubes). (**S/P**) A recommendation should be given that (medical) attention should be sought if the lid condition does not show signs of improvement within a few days.

(**b**) polymyxin B. This antibiotic inserts itself into bacterial membranes and makes them leaky to ions, especially Na^+ and H^+, and especially in gram positive bacteria causing lid infections and is used in combination with bacitracin. It is available as PoM **Polyfax**[R] (4 g tube; not approved for use by optometrists). Gramicidin is drug that exerts similar actions to polymyxin B, in that it too permeabilises bacterial membranes. Gramicidin is used in combination products only (see below).

(**c**) bacitracin zinc. The drug, as its zinc salt, blocks synthesis of the cell walls of common gram positive bacteria, although the mechanism of this inhibition is very different from other cell wall synthesis inhibitors (e.g. penicillins). It is used in the UK with polymyxin B and / or neomycin, e.g.

is available as PoM **Polyfax**^R (4 g tube); not approved for optometric use). An eye drop product, PoM **Neosporin**^R (5 mL bottle) is also available and contains neomycin, polymyxin B and gramicidin and is more generally used for conjunctivitis and / or as a post-operative eye drop.

All of these preparations are generally intended for short-term use only, i.e. just a few days, maximum 7-10 days. The antibiotic therapies may be repeated at intervals.The lids should be cleansed (but not excessively) and then the ointments worked into the lid margin (with a sterile cotton bud applicator) and the eyedrops used if the bulbar conjunctiva is affected as well. Nightly and morning use of the ointments should resolve the condition promptly for although these drugs probably have little action on the bacteria inside the inflamed loci, they should stop the infection spreading; the lid cleansing (perhaps along with warm compress application for 5 to 10 min) should promote expression of the foci.

(**d**) erythromycin and silver nitrate. In cases of acute conjunctivitis and blepharitis in infants (e.g. *ophthalmia neonatorum*), such treatments should also be effective. However, a hospital may also elect to use in-house erythromycin 0.5 % ophthalmic ointments. This drug is also fairly broad spectrum and replaces the use of silver nitrate 1 % solutions (Crede's treatment). One or two days of treatment is all that is usually needed. Neither erythromycin or silver nitrate are marketed for general ophthalmic use in the UK.

MANAGEMENT OF CHRONIC INFECTIONS OF THE LIDS

Patients presenting with an occasional stye or other inflammatory infections of the eyelash follicles or accessory lacrimal glands can be readily to managed with simple ocular hygiene and ocular anti-bacterial drugs in ointment form (see above). Longer term or recurrent conditions can still be managed (under appropriate supervision) with these preparations (i.e. P **Brolene**^R or PoM **Polyfax**^R eye ointments) but others may be needed as well. In chronic conditions, therapies should be alternated, i.e. use one preparation for 2 weeks and then switch to another for 2 weeks and then back again; this greatly reduces the chance of resistance developing. Other ophthalmic antibiotic ointments may be needed as well in chronic conditions. Other drugs that are useful include -

(**e**) chlortetracycline. This was introduced in the 1950's, and is now only marketed in ointment form (e.g. (PoM **Aureomycin**^R, chlortetracycline HCl 1 %, 3.5 g tubes) and used for recurrent lid infections not responsive to other anti-bacterials. Not recommended for use in children. Oral tetracyclines such as chlortetracycline or tetracycline may also used for long term management of blepharitis. (**S/P**) Eyelid photosensitivity reactions can occur.

In cases of chronic infections of the eyelids and conjunctiva, or inclusion conjunctivitis (e.g. as caused by *Chlamydia*) can be managed with topical chlortetracycline (or erythromycin; pharmacy-prepared or specially imported) ophthalmic ointment, but oral tetracyclines such as doxycycline (e.g. PoM **Vibramycin**[R]) or azithromycin (PoM **Zithromax**[R]) is recommended. Alternatively, oral erythromycin (e.g. PoM **Ilosone**[R]) might be considered but there are large number of drug interactions to be considered. Treatment of chlamydia infections is best done via an STD clinic since systemic treatment is very important. Other causes of chronic infections of the eyelids and conjunctiva include ocular rosacea and this condition may also be responsive to topical chlortetracycline and prolonged treatment with oral tetracyclines such as doxycycline or minocycline (PoM **Minocin**[R] **MR**). Topical skin gels or creams containing the nitroimidazole antibiotic, metronidazole (e.g. PoM **Rozex**[R], 30 g tube) may be very useful to reduce the facial and peri-ocular skin problems but are <u>not</u> for ocular use.

MANAGEMENT OF VIRAL INFECTIONS OF THE EYE

Certain viral infections of the external eye can be managed easily and with very favorable outcome, providing a prompt and correct diagnosis and the appropriate referral is made so that therapy is instigated and adhered to. In considering viral infections, the differential diagnosis is very important.

Patient history is very important. The <u>onset</u> of the condition tends to be acute for HSV and EKC (adenovirus) but subacute for HZ (varicella zoster). The <u>initial / early symptoms</u> and signs for HSV include foreign body sensation, annoying itching, tingling or moderate jabbing pain accompanied by lacrimation and photophobia are more likely; these are the classic signs and symptoms of a viral infection of the eye. For EKC however, slight irritation and itching accompanied by profuse lacrimation is more common while for HZ, itching (perhaps associated with tenderness of the eyelid and periocular skin), as well as involuntary twitching or phantom painful sensation are more common. HSV is the one more likely to present with a watery red eye. The <u>objective early signs</u> on examination will likely be distinctly different. For HSV, corneal positive staining with fluorescein or rose bengal may be punctate initially (especially in infant cases). These are very small foci of infected cells, and these discrete areas can later coalesce to form linear and branched patterns (dendrites). Corneal sensitivity may be reduced if it is a recurrent episode. For EKC, possible superficial punctate keratitis (that stains with fluorescein) or the appearance of subepithelial discrete opacities (that are non-staining) is more commonly encountered. A marked watery discharge and distinct follicular conjunctivitis may accompany the corneal signs, but this can occur with HSV, EKC and *Chlamydia* however. For HZ, early onset pseudo-dendritic (feathery) corneal patterns may be evident that may stain positively with fluorescein or rose bengal. Such signs are usually preceded by pain especially for the eyelid skin or peri-ocular / facial skin (and eruptions that are minute, focal or diffuse may be present on the skin). The eyelid margins may also be affected with cystic inclusions and encrustations. In later stages, HZ may resemble HSV in that the effects on the eye are more substantial in terms of symptoms with photophobia and the eye feels achy due to persistent lacrimation. With a unique coarse muco-purulent discharge, corneal patterns (pseudodendrites) may actually be mucous plaques that can change in size shape and position on the cornea on a daily basis. The removal of these plaques may be painful and the underlying area will now stain with rose bengal. At later stages, signs and symptoms can generally be expected to be rather different. For HSV, if significant epithelial erosion has occurred (i.e. there were substantial dendrites), infiltrating keratitis can develop into the stroma and can develop after the epithelial involvement has subsided. Due to reduction in corneal sensation there is usually less pain and photophobia than in other stromal infiltrates. For EKC, the condition should resolve to a quiet eye, despite residual epithelial or subepithelial deposits. For HZ, disciform keratitis of the anterior corneal stroma can develop that can be moderately painful.

Management of epidemic keratoconjunctivitis (EKC)

EKC is not generally indicated for treatment with anti-viral drugs. Management includes use of eye baths and topical ocular decongestants (e.g. naphazoline) *p.r.n.* (to reduce lacrimation and promote ocular comfort) and possible use of mild corticosteroid therapy to reduce the further development of corneal epithelial infiltrates. Such corticosteroid therapy should be q 6 h and usually only needs medium efficacy drugs (e.g. clobetasone 0.1 %). Steroid use should be tapered after 7 days. General hygiene measures to reduce the risk of cross-infection of other individuals is extremely important (including in the optometric office!) although they are not always effective (especially at home). The total treatment period is not usually more than 2 weeks.

Management of herpes simplex infections (HSV)

HSV should best receive prompt management with anti-viral drugs and care should be taken to prevent infection of other eye if the condition is unilateral (as it often is). Ophthalmic antiviral drugs work by blocking the ability of the virus to replicate DNA. They are mostly examples of pro-drugs in that the actual drug is largely ineffective against viruses but will be biotransformed by virus-infected epithelial cells into the active form of the drug (their triphosphorylated derivatives, e.g. aciclovir triphosphate). Regardless of the severity of presenting signs, therapy should be initiated with aciclovir 3 % ophthalmic ointment (PoM **Zovirax**^{R}, 4.5 g tube; expensive !). The dosing should be q 2 h or q 3 h, especially for the first 24h at which time the regimen could be reduced to q 4 h. Such a treatment should maintained for 7 days only, and preferably with examinations on days 1, 3 and 7. If, at 7 days, significant improvement and re-epithelialisation is underway, the dosing can be maintained at q 4 h for a further 3 to 5 days and then discontinued, i.e. it is important that therapy be continued for a few days after resolution is clearly underway. Treatment, if diagnosed early, should not need to be continued for more than 14 days.

Aciclovir preparations are also available as Pharmacy Medicines (e.g. P **Zovirax**[R] **Cold Sore Cream**, P **Herpetad**[R] or P **Soothelip**[R]). These are not for ophthalmic use, although may be indicated for topical skin use when the eye infections are associated with mouth ulcers or other skin lesions.

Another ophthalmic antiviral drug is trifluridine (also known as trifluorothymidine) but is only available via select hospital pharmacies in the UK (by special import), for severe cases of HSV keratitis. This drug is usually used as a 1 % solution and is widely used (as prescription-only VIROPTIC[R]) in North America. The regimen for use is intensive (e.g. q 1 h for 24 to 48 h) and then the frequency of use can be progressively reduced over several days to q 3 h. Seven to ten days therapy is usually all that is needed, and the drug should not be used much over this time period because of the risk of toxic effects to the corneal and conjunctival epithelium.

Another anti-viral drug for ophthalmic use was idoxuridine, but there are currently no marketed products in the UK. Its principal use in recent years was in milder and recurrent HSV infections wherein therapy could be initiated with idoxuridine 0.5 % ophthalmic ointment (PoM **Idoxene**[R], 3 g tube). Here, the regimen was q 4 h, with last application before bedtime. The patient still needed to be examined regularly to ensure that the condition did not develop further, and that re-epithelialisation was occurring. This option is now rarely used because of declining responsiveness of HSV infections to the idoxuridine. The ointment would need to be specially obtained from a hospital pharmacy. Treatment with idoxuridine ointment for more than 14 days was not recommended.

If the HSV infection, at presentation, is severe, other therapeutic measures need to be considered, including the systemic administration of anti-viral drugs such as aciclovir (PoM **Zovirax**[R] tablets). One other measure is to prompt recovery from the HSV infection by removing the virus- infected corneal epithelial cells before beginning anti-viral therapy, i.e. performing debridement. This is accomplished after intense topical anesthesia (e.g. several drops of amethocaine 0.5 %, or an ophthalmologist in a hospital may chose to use cocaine 4 % eye drops) followed by scraping the epithelium off with a surgical blade, or rubbing it off with a cotton bud applicator or a surgical spear. In deep, but focal dendritic figures, the epithelium may need to be scraped off around the lesion to promote re-epithelialisation. The primary goal in this measure (and the ensuing anti-viral therapy with acyclovir ointments) is to eradicate the virus as quickly as possible. The intensive use of the ointment containing anti-viral drugs may however retard epithelial re-surfacing and this needs to be carefully looked for during biomicroscopy in follow-up visits. In more serious infections, after an initial intensive topical anti-viral treatment (e.g. q 2 h for 24 to 36 h), the deep lesions (that may actually also involve the corneal stroma) might be carefully managed with strong topical ocular corticosteroids (e.g. PoM

Maxidex^R or PoM **Pred Forte**^{R}, *q.d.s.*) providing the patient can be seen on a daily basis (for a thorough slit lamp exam) to ensure that there is no further progression of the dendritic / infiltrating ulcers and that corneal resurfacing is well in progress. In such cases, IOP's should be recorded as well and pupil dilation / cycloplegia is also recommended to offset the iritis and flare that can develop in such cases (see below). With any indication of progression of the viral infection, the corticosteroid therapy should be promptly discontinued and intensive anti-viral therapy reinstituted.

<u>Management of herpes zoster (shingles) infections of the eye</u>

There are really two options here because it is not always easy to identify a zoster infection and it may be treated as an HSV infection initially or concurrently.

(i) for milder cases of HZ and where it is fairly certain that HSV is not present, it should be treated as an inflammatory condition (e.g. PoM **Maxidex**^{R}, PoM **Pred Forte**^{R} or PoM **Betnesol**^{R} eye drops *q.d.s.*) perhaps with an antibiotic eye drops (e.g. PoM **Garamycin**^{R}) after removal of the epithelial plaques by rubbing. Follow-up examination should be every 24 h for a few days to ensure that further infection does not develop. This topical treatment should best be accompanied by <u>oral anti-viral drugs</u> since zoster is generally a systemic infection. Current options include oral aciclovir (PoM **Zovirax**^{R}, 3 to 5 x 200 mg / day), oral famciclovir (PoM **Famvir**^{R}, 3 x 250 mg / day) or oral valaciclovir (PoM **Valtrex**^{R}, 2 x 500 mg, *t.d.s.*). The oral therapies will usually last 5-10 days. If further corneal dendrites appear then the condition was probably accompanied by HSV in which cases specific topical anti-viral measures must be taken (e.g. PoM **Zovirax**^{R} ophthalmic ointment).

(ii) in more severe cases (with eyelid vesicles / pustules, general muco-purulent discharge and general encrustation), or if dendrites continue to develop, treat as if there was HSV present with aciclovir ophthalmic ointment (see above). Pseudo-dendrites (plaques) removal should be attempted but debridement is not usually performed, since it is not as successful in such cases. Moderate-to-intensive steroid therapy is appropriate providing the patient can be seen every 24 to 48 h until the condition is clearly resolving. The steroid regimen must control the stromal involvement, BUT without worsening the condition by delaying re-epithelialisation or facilitating a secondary bacterial (or fungal) infection. The ophthalmic corticosteroid therapy may need to be continued for many weeks to many months. <u>Corticosteroid - antibiotic</u> therapy can also be considered. <u>Mydriatic - cycloplegic</u> treatment is essential (see chapter 17). As with milder cases, the topical therapies should be accompanied with <u>oral</u> anti-viral drugs (see above). <u>Systemic corticosteroids</u> (e.g. oral prednisolone 5 mg tablets X 8, in divided doses) may be needed (PoM **Deltacortril**; numerous generic products available).

The use of cold compresses, adjunct use of artificial tears and even topical ocular decongestants may provide much needed symptomatic relief for discomfort / pain, along with milder oral analgesics (e.g. G **Paracodol**[R], paracetamol 500 mg with codeine 8 mg or equivalent) *vs.* strong oral narcotic analgesics (e.g. CD **Pethidine**[R], pethidine 50 to 150 mg *t.d.*s.). Some have also recommended that the pain of facial zoster lesions can be managed with a special topical (skin) analgesic preparations containing a compound called capsaicin [*cap-say-sin*] (e.g. PoM **Axsain**[R] 0.075 % cream, PoM **Zacin**[R] 0.025 % cream) either on its own, or as a supplement to the oral narcotic analgesics. Weaker preparations containing a related compound capsicum (e.g GSL **Balmosa**[R] cream) are not recommended because other ingredients may aggravate the skin lesions.

MANAGEMENT OF FUNGAL INFECTIONS OF THE EYE

Relatively few specific anti-fungal drugs exist and even fewer are specifically indicated for use in ocular infections caused by fungi and protozoa, let alone actually being indicated for topical ocular use, i.e. fungal infections of the external eye are not really the realm of topical therapy. The management of these infections will be discussed here because there is always a risk with any bacterial or viral infection that inappropriate diagnosis or therapy will result in opportunistic infection with fungi or protozoa.

Fungal infections are almost invariably well progressed and very severe by the time a diagnosis is made. As a result, any anti-infective medications that are then used are always going to be working against the odds and may need to be used for extended periods (i.e. weeks to months) rather than just a few days to a couple of weeks as for bacterial or viral infections. Therapy of ocular fungal or protozoan infections is thus managed by the specialist even though, in many cases, there is little that can be done for such infections and the prognosis for even some reasonable vision after intensive therapy is generally poor. However, and especially nowadays, medical therapy is being tried more and more and in the hope that an eye can be saved or, perhaps, be prevented from deteriorating to a full and out-of-control general infection. To illustrate these infections, the therapy and strategies for an infection caused by fungi (*Candida, Fusarium,* or *Aspergillus*) will be covered.

Most fungal infections of the external eye and anterior segment are usually diagnosed as viral infections, and then initially managed as viral infections. This is simply because the signs (acute or sub-acute red eye, lacrimation, little or no discharge) and symptoms (marked foreign body sensation, moderate pain and photophobia) resemble those of an HSV infection. There may even be discrete punctate staining of the epithelium and central sub-epithelial infiltrates, and dendrite-like figures or infiltrates have also been reported. However linear infiltrates (even railway track-like infiltrates that may or may not follow the path of the more superficial corneal nerves) can also be present and these may be a distinguishing early sign that there is a fungal or protozoan infection.

A fungal (or protozoan) infection be suspected IF there is a failure of such a red eye to show some positive response to anti-bacterial or anti-viral therapy (usually with modest supplementary anti-inflammatory therapy) within 3 to 4 weeks of regular therapy. As a general rule, any infection of the external eye that does not respond well to such therapy should be assumed to be fungal or protozoan until proven otherwise and appropriate measures taken. This requires aggressive management that includes the collection of conjunctival or epithelial scrapings (under topical anesthesia) for diagnostic purposes and cultures. Unusually high levels of ocular pain are a further indicator of a fungal or protozoan infection, i.e. the red eye hurts much more than its external appearance suggests. The reason is perhaps the association of the infective organisms with the corneal nerves. The diagnosis will be, in part, made on the detection of fungal hyphae in scrapings from the ocular surface or, for example, in a patient's contact lens cases, e.g. those due to organisms such as *Candida, Fusarium* or *Aspergillus*. Treatments can only be done via a major hospital centre since the ophthalmic drugs need to be prepared by a pharmacy. Drug therapies include -

(**a**) topical anti-fungal drugs, e.g. natamycin 3 % or 5 % ophthalmic suspension. This suspension can be prepared by a hospital pharmacy from a powder and a suitable vehicle (or a major hospital may have a special arrangement to use a commercial product from the USA, prescription-only NATACYN[R]). If hospital-prepared, the natamycin suspension is best stored in a 4°C refrigerator once prepared. For fungal keratitis, treatment should be *q* 1 h for 3 to 4 days, day and night. Thereafter the dosing can perhaps be reduced to *q* 2 h or to *q* 3h. Less intense therapies could be used for fungal conjunctivitis or blepharitis. Since the fungal infection is not usually accompanied by substantial exudative signs (discharge etc.), the reduction of dosing after 3 to 4 days will also provide an indication of whether the organism is being controlled. If some improvement is not observed in 7 to 10 days, then the causative organism is not likely to be a susceptible fungus. The treatment period, for resolution, is normally 14 to 28 days if responsive but more established cases may require several weeks therapy.

(**b**) topical corticosteroids. Controversial and difficult clinical decision. At some point after initiation of the anti-fungal topical therapy, a decision has to be made to add topical corticosteroid therapy. The earliest should be 4 days, but the main point is that the corticosteroid therapy should only be started when the fungus infection is clearly under control. The corticosteroid therapy is essential if scarring of the corneal tissue is to kept to a minimum and is also required to promote recovery of the tissue from the substantial edema that can develop. Corticosteroid therapy has to approached carefully since the corticosteroid use could exacerbate the fungal invasion of the corneal and conjunctival tissue; moderate dosing (e.g. *q* 4 h or *q* 6 h) with stronger corticosteroid preparations (PoM **Maxidex**[R] eye drops or PoM **Pred Forte**[R] eye drops etc.) should be sufficient.

(**c**) other antifungal eye drops, e.g. amphotericin B [*am-fo-ter-ee-sin*]. In rare cases, the initial condition is already severe, or an identified fungal infection (based on scrapings and cultures) continues to worsen despite natamycin treatment. In such types of cases, and only for these, an alternative treatment could be with specially prepared amphotericin B eye drops. This drug is primarily marked as an anti-fungal for *i.v.* use (PoM **Fungizone**[R]) but the powder can be reconstituted in sterile water to make eye drops. Once the amphotericin eye drops are prepared, they should be very carefully protected from light at all times. Furthermore, if a refrigerator is not available all the time, the eye drops should be discarded each day and a new bottle started. If a refrigerator is available, the drops could be used for a week. A concentration of just 1 mg/mL (i.e. 0.1 %) is recommended because the drug is very toxic. The initial regimen would be something like *q* 30 min to *q* 1 h for 2 to 3 days, day and night, then the dosing frequency can be reduced to *q* 1 h *q* 2 h etc. at daily intervals. The solution is likely to be toxic to the cornea and conjunctiva, so the period of treatment should not be extended beyond 7 to 10 days.

NOTE. Adjunct therapies should also include topical corticosteroids, cycloplegics and narcotic analgesics, and oral anti-fungal drugs if the ocular infection is associated with skin or mucous membrane infections with the same fungus.

MANAGEMENT OF PROTOZOAN INFECTIONS OF THE EYE

The example chosen here is that caused by *Acanthamoeba* sp., and the types of treatment detailed are meant to illustrate the types of multiple therapies that will be simultaneously used in such infections. There is no fixed treatment for such infections neither are there specific regimens that have been rigorously evaluated. Such therapies represent a series of last-stage measures to try to save a cornea and the eye and the prognosis is never good. It is likely that the types of therapy outlined below will need to be continued for at least 3 months, and perhaps even 6 or 9 months!. At some point, consideration needs to be given to the use of topical ocular corticosteroids to manage the edema and inflammation but always at the risk of exacerbating the protozoan infection.

Following diagnosis based on history (see above) or conjunctival or corneal scrapings showing the presence of cysts, therapies that have been tried include -

(**a**) instigate *intensive* therapy with propamidine 0.1 % eye drops (i.e. P **Brolene**[R], or P **Golden Eye**[R] eye drops) *q* 30 min for 1 day, then *q* 1 h on second day, then *q* 2 h thereafter until there is some response; this should only be done under hospital supervision. Thereafter, the regimen may be reduced, e.g. to *q* 4h. This is obviously a special and extraordinary use of propamidine eye drops and not one that was even known about when these eye drops were initially introduced for management of mild bacterial infections of the lids and conjunctiva (see above). It should be stressed that this type of use of propamidine eye drops is definitely not to be instigated under anything other than very close medical supervision. The ointments may be used at night in later stages of the therapy.

Currently, an alternative to propamidine that is has been tried at some hospital specialist eye clinics is to use a hospital-pharmacy prepared 0.2 % solution of chlorhexidine on a similarly intensive regimen to propamidine; eye drops of other "preservatives" are also being evaluated. As with propamidine therapies, management of a contact lens-wear -related "red eye" should <u>not</u> be attempted with commercial lens disinfecting solutions, no matter how intense the regimen of use.

(**b**) start concurrent intensive therapy with a <u>broad spectrum anti-bacterial</u>, e.g. <u>fortified</u> gentamicin 1 % eye drops, *q* 2 h or more frequently. The fortified gentamicin will be prepared by a major hospital pharmacy. The anti-bacterial therapy is considered useful since the "sterilisation" of the ocular surface should reduce any possible replication of the amoebae (that feed on bacteria). In later stages of the therapy, a combination antibiotic therapy (e.g. PoM **Neosporin**[R] eyedrops) may be used instead, but still on an intensive regimen.

(**c**) use an <u>oral anti-infective</u> (imidazole type) drug such as ketoconazole, 200 to 400 mg *q.d.* (e.g. PoM **Nizoral**[R], *tab*). This can be used concurrently with the propamidine eye drops since this "anti-fungal" has some effect on protozoan plasma membranes as well and can be protozoocidal at high doses. However, such drugs are much less effective against the cyst forms of *Acanthamoeba*.

Additional measures include intensive topical <u>cycloplegic</u> therapy and oral analgesics, especially <u>narcotic</u> <u>analgesics</u>.

OPHTHALMIC ANTI-BACTERIAL - CORTICOSTEROID COMBINATIONS.

Purpose of chapter. In some diseases of the external eye (including the lids), a significant inflammatory response accompanies an infection, principally by bacteria. In other diseases, there is an inflammation that leaves the ocular surface compromised and at risk for infection. In both types of situation, combination (simultaneous) therapy using ophthalmic corticosteroid drugs with anti-bacterial drugs is indicated either short term, medium term or even longer term. In some situations, therapy could require the addition of a corticosteroid to an anti-bacterial regimen, or could require the addition of an anti-bacterial drug to an ongoing corticosteroid regimen. There has traditionally been uncertainty and controversy in the use of these combinations and either extreme has been acceptable at different periods of time, i.e. either that combination therapy is the superior mode of therapy, or that combination therapy is not only ineffective but considered dangerous. It is the goals of this chapter to outline the options that are available and to consider the reasons for and against this type of therapy, and the patient management that is required.

Indications for concurrent anti-infective/ corticosteroid therapy

For commonly encountered conditions, there are really three reasons why combination therapy with anti-bacterial drugs and corticosteroids may be considered -

(**a**) for short-term management of inflammatory disease associated with bacterial infections of the external eye.

(**b**) for chronic, mild-to-moderate, inflammation of the anterior segment of the eye where there is a risk of bacterial infection, or a bacterial infection is actually present. Such conditions can range from cases of severe allergic conjunctivitis, blepharo-conjunctivitis, vernal conjunctivitis, acne rosacea and select cases of episcleritis. Some cases of non-specific toxic keratitis may also respond well to such combination therapy.

(**c**) for moderate-to-severe inflammatory conditions of the anterior segment where intensive corticosteroid therapy is essential, but there is a real risk of bacterial infection (e.g. herpes zoster infections, post-trauma keratitis from burns, chemical injuries, significant post-operative keratitis or after the removal of deep or penetrating foreign bodies, or following many types of ocular surgery).

This type of combination therapy is controversial and so it can be expected that it will be approached cautiously, and also require some extra patient management. There are a number of general issues that should be considered *before* use of anti-bacterial-corticosteroid combination products.

(**a**) (**S/P**) corticosteroid therapies will do nothing to combat a bacterial infection in terms of slowing bacterial replication or preventing their spread. The opposite has in fact been argued in that concurrent corticosteroid therapy may exacerbate an infection (partly because the corticosteroids may mask the ongoing development of the infection).

(**b**) (**S/P**) longer term steroid use increases the risk of overgrowth of pathogens that are non-responsive to anti-bacterial drugs. These include both resistant strains of bacteria, opportunistic bacteria as well as fungi etc. The risk is present partly because the corticosteroid therapy masks the development of a secondary infection.

(**c**) (**S/P**) excessive or inappropriate corticosteroid use may cause diseases of the ocular surface. The corticosteroid use may slow the rate of re-epithelialization and / or promote destabilization of the ocular surface, especially when there is an infection present. The epithelium is the best natural barrier against infection and so its re-formation is an essential part of managing diseases of the ocular surface.

(**d**) (**C/I**) steroid use is contraindicated when active HSV, fungal or protozoan keratitis is present, or there is active Tb infection. Steroid use should also be very carefully monitored when there is a substantial bacterial infection present (for reasons explained above).

CORTICOSTEROIDS ADDED TO ANTI-BACTERIAL THERAPY

Typical examples here would include chronic cases of blepharitis or blepharo-conjunctivitis, secondary management of moderate-to-severe bacterial infections of the conjunctiva and cornea. In practical terms, several simple issues should be considered -

(**a**) Patient comfort. The added corticosteroid therapy is designed to improve patient comfort and to promote recovery from inflammatory consequences of the infection, while still maintaining coverage against the bacteria. If anti-bacterial therapy was simply switched to a corticosteroid therapy (to reduce the consequences of the infection), the bacterial infection may flare up again. Patient comfort is promoted because any degree of resolution of tissue oedema will reduce the "puffy eye" sensation as well as reduce pain. The recovery from inflammation is promoted because the corticosteroids should reduce the leakiness of the vasculature and thus stem the ongoing extravasation process. For lid conditions, the corticosteroid therapy should reduce invasion of the conjunctival epithelium and the underlying stroma by white blood cells to promote optimum restoration of the natural architecture of these very important surfaces. Without corticosteroid therapies, and especially in recurrent infections, scarring of the tissue may result in poor lid closure (with long term consequences in terms of maintaining a normal tear film). For corneal conditions, the corticosteroid use is designed to limit the extent of white blood cell migration into the corneal tissue to promote optimum visual outcome, i.e. avoid corneal scars.

(**b**) the steroid selection and the dose administered should be able to effectively keep the inflammation under control. This is important, for while overdosing with the corticosteroids could lead to exacerbation of the condition, under-dosing could mean that the inflammatory condition is not effectively controlled which means that the steroid therapy is of questionable value. The longer the external tissues of the eye are inflamed, the greater the chance of opportunistic infections.

(**c**) the corticosteroid dosing regimen only needs to be continued for as long as the inflammation is considered to be significant enough to need such anti-inflammatory drug therapy. Once the inflammation is under control, the corticosteroid dosing can be reduced and this is best done by progressively tapering the corticosteroid dose. This will most commonly be done by simply reducing the frequency of administration of the combination pharmaceutical. Since the corticosteroid was added to a condition wherein the bacterial infection was already controlled, the progressive reduction in dosing frequency is also compatible with the expected status of the infection. Such tapering of the corticosteroid therapy will improve reliability of assessments of the severity of the lid, conjunctival or corneal condition.

(**d**) (**S/P**) On lowering steroid dose, and on especially upon discontinuation of the corticosteroid therapy, signs and symptoms may get a little worse for a day or so especially if there is still a mild degree of infection still present. Should this occur, it should be the anti-bacterial therapy that is intensified, not the corticosteroid.

(**e**) (**ADR**) Any ophthalmic corticosteroid therapy requires consideration of IOP if the treatment is for more than 1 to 2 weeks. Ideally, IOP's should be known before any ophthalmic corticosteroid therapy is started. In the presence of a conjunctival or corneal bacterial infection, IOP may already be slightly elevated (by 3 to 5 mm Hg). Any patient may show an unusual progressive elevation of IOP, especially following longer-term therapy with corticosteroid-containing eyedrops; regular IOP monitoring is thus essential (e.g. every 10 to 14 days where appropriate). Some corticosteroid-containing eyedrops (e.g. those with hydrocortisone or dexamethasone) are considered more likely to raise IOP than the other steroids. However when a compromised epithelium is present, it would be better to assume that any topical ophthalmic corticosteroid could raise IOP over 2 to 4 weeks.

(**e**) (**ADR**) Consideration of any other corticosteroid-induced adverse drug reactions. Patients who have a history of recurrent inflammations associated with infections of the eye and who have had intermittent treatment with ophthalmic corticosteroids, should be monitored for cataract formation, especially PSSC (see chapter 11). Some have advocated that, for such patients, ophthalmic corticosteroid therapies of longer than 3 weeks in duration should only be managed by an ophthalmologist.

ANTI-BACTERIALS ADDED TO CORTICOSTEROID THERAPY

Other cases for combination therapy can be prompted by a need to provide anti-bacterial coverage for an eye that is being managed with corticosteroids and usually on a longer term basis. For such therapies -

(**a**) coverage with anti-bacterials should be approached as being a temporary measure to reduce the chance of infection in a chronically irritated and inflamed eye.

(**b**) in considering the dosing with anti-bacterials, it should be recognized that the steroids may significantly mask usual signs and symptoms associated with a bacterial eye infection and so it is better to err on the excess side rather than under-dose with the required anti-bacterials. From the corticosteroid perspective, such combination therapies should be conservative, not intensive, due to the masking effects and consideration should even be given to slightly reducing the corticosteroid therapy while anti-bacterial coverage is provided. If the infection really flares up, corticosteroid therapy should be discontinued and intensive anti-bacterial therapy initiated.

(**c**) this use of combination products always carries a higher risk than that the corticosteroid-masking of the signs and symptoms could lead to misdiagnosis of the infection.

(**d**) more attention should be paid to follow-up so that corticosteroid therapy can be discontinued (and anti-bacterial therapy intensified) if an infection develops or gets worse. Equally importantly, the anti-bacterial drug use should only be continued for as long as is necessary to control infection and, after the eye is quiet again (e.g. no muco-purulent discharge etc.), the anti-bacterial drug should be discontinued. Over-use of the anti-bacterial drugs could result in the development of unwanted resistance to the anti-bacterial drugs.

AVAILABLE COMBINATION PRODUCTS AND THEIR USE

The following recommendations are based on the premise that the use matched drugs and of a line of products from one source is easier than mixing drugs or sources. Since consideration is being given primarily to temporarily adding a corticosteroid to an anti-bacterial regimen being used in moderate-to severe infections, practical product options are listed by anti-bacterial drug and grouped by commercial product lines where appropriate:-

(a) chloramphenicol. An ointment combination product was available until mid-1996, but its current availability (for human use) use is questionable (e.g. PoM **Chloromycetin - Hydrocortisone**[R], 4 g tubes). The combination can obviously also be achieved by combining hydrocortisone 1 % eye drops (PoM **Hydrocortisone**, generic) or 0.5 or 1 % ophthalmic ointment (PoM **Hydrocortisone**, generic) with chloramphenicol 0.5 % eye drops (e.g. PoM **Sno-Phenicol**[R], 10 mL bottle) or 1 % ointment (e.g. PoM **Chloromycetin**[R], or PoM **Chloramphenicol Eye Ointment** BP, both 4 g tubes). With hydrocortisone being only a moderate strength corticosteroid, the use of these combination product would best be limited to lid and conjunctival conditions requiring this type of therapy. These products, with chloramphenicol, should not be used if the conditions are recurrent because of a special risk of patient sensitization to chloramphenicol with ensuring risk development of ADR's (see chapter 14). Combination therapy should be continued until the inflammation resolves, and then the use of the combination product tapered to *o.d.* (or the ointment combination being used *o.n.*) and therapy with the anti-bacterial continued for two or three more days. The ointment could also be used on a *q.d.s.* basis until the inflammation was managed, and then the use of the product tapered.

(b) framycetin. A companion corticosteroid product is available that contains framycetin 0.5 % and gramicidin 0.005 % with dexamethasone 0.05 % (PoM **Sofradex**[R]; eyedrops 10 mL and eye ointment 5 g). The combination could also be achieved with framycetin 0.5 % eye drops (10 mL bottle) or ointment (5 g tube) (both PoM **Soframycin**[R]), and dexamethasone 0.1 % eye drops (PoM **Maxidex**[R]). The dexamethasone is expected to be a strong corticosteroid product and should promptly resolve any inflammation. These types of product could therefore be used to manage lid, conjunctival and corneal infectious inflammations. The use of the eye drops would usually be *q.d.s,.* with the ointment being used nightly (*o.n.*), perhaps only along with the use of the anti-bacterial eye drops during the day instead of the combination product being used during the day. Combination therapy should be continued until the inflammation resolves and then the use of the combination product tapered to *o.d.* (or the ointment combination being used *o.n.*) and then simply discontinued. The treatment with the anti-bacterial product should be continued for 2 or 3 more days.

(c) neomycin is available for this wide spectrum of uses in combination with weak corticosteroids (e.g. PoM **Neo-Cortef**[R], neomycin 0.5 % with hydrocortisone acetate 1.5 %, 5 mL, 10 mL bottles and 3.9 g ointment tubes), with low concentrations of moderate strength corticosteroids (e.g. PoM **Maxitrol**[R], neomycin 0.35 % plus polymyxin B 6000 units / mL with dexamethasone 0.1 %, 5 mL bottles, 3.5 g tubes), with low concentrations of steroids (e.g. PoM **FML - Neo**[R], neomycin 0.5 % with fluorometholone 0.1 %, 5 mL bottles only), with higher concentrations of corticosteroids (e.g. PoM **Predsol-N**[R], neomycin 0.5 % with prednisolone 0.5 %, 10 mL bottles only) and finally with strong steroids (e.g. PoM **Betnesol-N**[R], neomycin 0.5 % with betamethasone 0.1 %, 10 mL bottles *or* PoM **Vista-Methasone**[R], neomycin 0.5 % with betamethasone 0.1 %, 5 mL and 10 mL bottles). A combination with clobetasone (PoM **Cloburate-N**[R], 10 mL bottles only) was discontinued in early 1998. Neomycin itself is available as unit dose (PoM **Minims**[R] **Neomycin**, 0.5 %) and widely available as generics (PoM **Neomycin**, drops and ointments). With the numerous combination products neomycin being available, neomycin - corticosteroid products are probably those most commonly used for management of infections of the lids, conjunctiva and cornea that require some anti-inflammatory drug therapy (as well as standard post-operative drugs for ocular surgery). Optometric use of neomycin-containing products is not approved. Those products that are ointments are those that are more likely to be used for management of infections of the lids and conjunctiva where some anti-inflammatory drug cover is required as well. For such products, the use of the combination eye drops would usually be *q.d.s.* with the ointment being used nightly (perhaps only along with the use of the anti-bacterial eye drops during the day instead of the combination product being used during the day). Combination therapy should be continued until the inflammation resolves and then the use of the combination product tapered to *o.d.* (or the ointment combination being used *o.n*) and therapy with the anti-bacterial continued for two or three more days. For their surgical use, only the eye drops are likely to be used (see below).

(**d**) gentamicin, fusidic acid, ciprofloxacin, ofloxacin, chlortetracycline and propamidine are not available as combination products in the UK although all of them can be used in combination with corticosteroids if appropriate; this would need to be done by prescribing a separate bottle of the corticosteroid eye drops in addition to the prescribed anti-bacterial eye drops. With the current indications for use of these anti-infective drugs for more serious infections or special cases, a potent corticosteroid product (e.g. PoM **Pred-Forte**[R]) would be the first choice for corticosteroid selection to be used concurrently with a suitable anti-bacterial product.

If an anti-bacterial drug is being added to corticosteroid therapy *or* included with corticosteroid therapy, then the same ophthalmic pharmaceuticals are going to be used but with a slightly different emphasis. In addition to chronic inflammations of the external eye, the commonest use for corticosteroids is as a standard post-operative treatment to counter the inflammation produced by the operation. In such cases, the anti-bacterial drug coverage is primarily prophylactic, i.e. to minimize the risk of post-operative eye infections. In these cases, the primary combination products that will be used with be those containing neomycin with moderate to strong corticosteroids (prednisolone or betamethasone) or framycetin with moderately strong corticosteroids (e.g. with dexamethasone).

ANTI-BACTERIAL CORTICOSTEROID THERAPIES WITH
MYDRIATIC / CYCLOPLEGIC USE

When inflammations of the eye develop, there are special uses of mydriatic-
cycloplegic drugs. Similarly, the use of mydriatic-cycloplegic drugs is part
of a normal standard of care for eyes considered at risk for developing
inflammation. Eyes with bacterial infections of the conjunctiva and cornea
(or many other types of infection), or considered at risk for bacterial
infections of the conjunctiva and cornea fall into categories for use of
mydriatic-cycloplegics. Such use is for two reasons. Firstly, their use is for
preventive care in acute, sub-acute or chronic intra-ocular inflammation
where adhesions may develop between the miotic pupil and the lens
capsule. The synechiae, if uncorrected, can lead to iris atrophy or damage
and this could be most unwanted, especially as a post-operative
complication. Even "plastic" intra-ocular lenses can adhere to an inflamed
iris. For patients with moderate-to-severe infectious inflammations of the
eye or as a standard post-operative treatment, the additional use of a
mydriatic-cycloplegic should promote patient comfort. Iritis or uveitis, etc.,
is often painful and sometimes extremely painful. Therapy with a mydriatic-
cycloplegic drug is essential to reduce this pain (perhaps with
supplementary systemic analgesics). The mydriatic-cycloplegics also
reduce vasodilatation of the inflamed tissues so can be expected to reduce
the development of oedema etc. The cycloplegic effects reduce the
"tugging" sensation that accompanies inflammation and spasms of muscle
contraction.

For these types of cases, the mydriatic-cycloplegic use is usually instigated
at either the first signs of intraocular inflammation associated with an
infection, or after any form of trauma to the eye (e.g. surgery). Therapy
should be continued for as long as the intra-ocular inflammation or risk of
inflammation is present. The following need to be considered -

(i) (S/P) physical characteristics of the anterior segment. The same type of
limitations that apply to the diagnostic use of mydriatic-cycloplegics also
apply to their therapeutic use. It can be noted however that while eyes with
"narrow angles" are at risk for angle closure, eyes that develop posterior
synechiae are at even greater risk of a secondary angle closure so the
benefits of the use of the mydriatic-cycloplegic to control inflammation
must be weighed against the other risks. Generally speaking, the benefit will
outweigh the risks, especially because IOP is likely to reduced during the
longer term course of intra-ocular inflammation.

(ii) pigmentation of the eye and pharmacokinetics of mydriatic-
cycloplegics. The extent of the cycloplegia is important for such therapies
and the dosing regimen chosen should be consistent with the degree of
ocular pigmentation, i.e. the darker the eye, the greater the dosing needed.

(**iii**) <u>extent of inflammation</u>. The mydriatic action serves to counter both the inflammation-related miosis (due to release of certain prostaglandins and substance P) and the inflammation-related contraction and oedema of the ciliary body. The use of the mydriatic-cycloplegic may only produce slight mydriasis (as opposed to the pupil being miotic) but can produce substantial mydriasis. Depending on patient age, proportionate changes in the amplitude of accommodation will occur as well. The goal is more to relax the muscles inside the eye, rather than try to achieve maximal effects.

(**iv**) <u>duration of the therapy</u> required. The duration of the treatment very much depends on the severity of the presenting signs and symptoms or the severity of the anticipated ocular response to the trauma, etc. For example, a few days of therapy would be appropriate for cases of acute infections and 1 to 2 weeks for anterior-segment surgery. The need for the mydriatic-cycloplegics will be dependent upon the extent of use of corticosteroids and *vice versa*.

(**vi**) <u>dosing recommendations</u> for therapeutic use of mydriatic-cycloplegics. The usual drug is atropine 1 %, i.e. PoM **Atropine** (generic) or PoM **Isopto Atropine**[R] eye drops, 10 mL or 5 mL bottles respectively; **Minims**[R] **Atropine Sulphate** (unit-dose eye drops) could be used for very short term management. The atropine should be used *o.d.* (mild -to-moderate cases), *b.d.s* (moderate-to-severe cases) or *q.d.s* (very severe cases). A generic **Atropine** 1 % ointment can be used *o.d.* (preferably *o.n.*). If the eyes are darkly (as opposed to lightly) pigmented, minimal therapy should be *b.d.s.* but greater than *q.d.s.* dosing should not be needed even for severe cases in darkly-pigmented eyes since the cycloplegic effects will persist with the repeated applications. As a practical note, the cycloplegic should be the last of the drops instilled into the eye at a dosing time since these eye drops tend to sting more than others; reflex tearing will wash the antibacterial / corticosteroid drugs out from the eye thus reducing the efficacy. A 5 to 10 minute interval, between antibiotic / corticosteroid eye drops and the mydriatic-cycloplegic, is reasonable.

Some practitioners prefer the use of homatropine as a therapeutic cycloplegic but the available multiple-use pharmaceuticals only contain 1 % or 2 % homatropine, rather than 5 % (e.g. PoM **Homatropine** eye drops; generic, 10 mL bottles) and so are really only for moderate cases and should be used at least *b.d.s*; a PoM **Minims**[R] **Homatropine Hydrobromide** (unit-dose) is available at the 2 % concentration but really only for very short term management. Hyoscine 0.25 % (e.g.PoM **Hyoscine**, generic; 10 mL bottle) can also be used as an alternative to homatropine in moderate-to-severe cases, again at a minimum *b.i.d.* regimen. These drug doses and regimens are necessary since the pharmacokinetics of these drugs are substantially. different in the inflamed eye compared to the un-inflamed eye.

(S/P) <u>Patient follow-up</u>. Periodic checks (e.g. every 2 to 3 weeks for longer term therapies) need to be carried out both for general examination of the eye and also for IOP assessments. The periodic check ups are especially important to check for symptoms and signs of systemic atropine "poisoning", especially in very young or elderly debilitated patients. This should be done more frequently if corticosteroids are also administered and / or the patient has a history of (or is considered at risk for) development of moderate to substantially elevated IOP (see chapter 18).

PRE- AND POST-SURGICAL USE of NON-STEROIDAL ANTI-INFLAMMATORY DRUGS

The use of corticosteroids and cycloplegics as standard post-operative drugs in cataract surgery has been much reduced in recent years with the use of topical ophthalmic non-steroidal anti-inflammatory drugs, both before and after surgery. These drugs have both a general anti-inflammatory action and can have a unique analgesic action.

Traditionally, the use of anti-inflammatory drugs on the eye has been promoted whenever there was evidence of the possible development of inflammatory signs, when clear signs of inflammation were present, or the eye had been subject to a form of trauma (especially chemical or mechanical, including surgery) where inflammation was an expected sequel to the trauma. Such inflammation may be confined to the external eye or affect the anterior uvea, iris or vitreous and retina. The non-steroidal anti-inflammatory drugs (NSAID's) serve to counteract the inflammatory process *per se* and thus can also be considered as a true therapy for at least some aspects of the inflammatory response. By reducing the tissue production of a group of vasodilators called prostaglandins, these drugs can be very effectively used prophylactically, i.e. prior to and in anticipation of the inflammation. It seems very likely that numerous NSAID's will be developed for extraocular use the next few years. To date, every currently-used systemic NSAID has been tested in laboratory or pre-clinical trials for their efficacy in a large number of ocular conditions (mild and severe). Such use extends a practice dating back to the 1890's that systemic acetylsalicylic acid (**Aspirin**[R]) could reduce the severity of ocular inflammation. In addition, several other NSAID's (although not currently marketed or used as systemic medications) have been evaluated for their efficacy in combatting various inflammatory conditions in the eye. To many people, NSAID is a term that is restricted to the many different types of "aspirin" - related drugs that serve to attenuate or inhibit a tissue enzyme called prostaglandin synthase; it is the activity of this enzyme that results in the production of prostaglandins. If the rate of prostaglandin production is slowed down, there should be an attenuation of the inflammatory reaction that follows trauma, etc. However, the NSAID term is becoming more widely applied in practice (rightly or wrongly) to include other drugs that indirectly reduce inflammation-related events. Therefore, any drug that might reduce vasodilatation (and the resultant vessel leakiness and tissue oedema that is so characteristic of seasonal or vernal conjunctivitis), might be considered as having NSAID-like actions. For this chapter, the term NSAID will however be restricted to the "aspirin"-like drugs.

(**i**) diclofenac sodium [*dye-kloh-fen-ak*] (PoM **Voltarol**^R **Ophtha**; do not confuse with other diclofenac products with the same brand name). This is a 0.1 % solution marketed in Unit-dose packages that has three uses. As a NSAID, it can reduce the risk of cystoid macular edema (CME) postoperatively for cataract patients. It also has been shown to be able to maintain mydriasis during surgery and is also considered to have sufficient anti-inflammatory efficacy to be used to manage general ocular inflammation (in addition to macular inflammation) after surgery. Its demonstrated efficacy at maintaining a dilated pupil intra-operatively is because it inhibits the prostaglandin production that can cause miosis (even in the presence of pre-operative mydriatics such as tropicamide with phenylephrine or cyclopentolate). Its efficacy in generally reducing inflammation of the eye means that, with its pre-operative use, less post-operative corticosteroid therapy is needed. The recommended use in surgical situations is to instill several drops into the eye in the time period shortly before surgery (i.e. over 2 to 3 hrs) and then use the drops 4 to 5 times day for as long as is necessary after surgery. This post-operative dosing period is probably 4 to 6 weeks for most patients. Diclofenac eye drops are also gaining popularity as a post-operative drug after laser surgery of the cornea. As well as reducing inflammation, diclofenac appears to have remarkable efficacy as a pain killer (analgesic) following these types of surgery (laser keratectomy etc.); this analgesic effect reduces the need for post-operative narcotic analgesics, and is a currently-approved indication for **Voltarol**^R **Ophtha**.

(**ii**) ketorolac trometamol ophthalmic solution (PoM **Acular**^R) 0.5 % is another NSAID, also only indicated as a prophylactic for inflammation and associated symptoms following cataract surgery. Its use is similar to diclofenac, e.g. *t.d.s.* for the day prior to surgery, and then *t.d.s.* for up to three weeks post-operatively.

(**iii**) flurbiprofen ophthalmic solution (PoM **Ocufen**^R). This is a 0.03 % solution in 1.4 % polyvinyl alcohol. It is only indicated for intensive use as a general anti-inflammatory drug for cataract operations, especially in cases where corticosteroids are contraindicated. It is marketed in Unit-dose packages. Recommended dosing is just before surgery (e.g. 1 *gtt q* 30 min for 2 h) and then *q* 4 h for 1 to 3 weeks after surgery.

SYSTEMIC DRUG INTERACTIONS WITH THE POSTERIOR SEGMENT (CRYSTALLINE LENS, INTRA-OCULAR PRESSURE, VISUAL ACUITY, VISUAL FIELDS and RETINAL APPEARANCE)

Purpose of chapter. The administration of even common medications can cause subtle changes in intra-ocular pressure (IOP) and thus an understanding of the potential for these types of changes and why they occur is very important for any interpretation of an IOP reading. In rarer cases, systemic drug interactions with the posterior part of the eye can cause changes in the crystalline lens (leading to a deterioration in vision), can cause secondary changes in retinal function (leading to altered vision or visual fields), can cause direct or indirect toxic effects on neural function (including that of the optic nerve) and be associated with dramatic changes in blood supply to the retina and optic nerve. In some cases, evidence suggests that the visual changes or the clinically measured changes can be reversible, so that prompt discontinuation of the drugs at the first sign of any problems may be very strongly recommended. In other cases, the extent (appearance) of the changes may appear substantial yet have little or no effects on VA or visual fields so careful monitoring is appropriate rather than discontinuing the drug therapy. Lastly, there are cases where these iatrogenic effects are substantial and affecting vision, yet it can still be argued that without the medication(s) the patients life-style or life expectancy would be so reduced that vision side effects are secondary (and an "unavoidable" consequence of the drug therapies). The goals of this chapter are therefore to summarize these drug interactions and provide some realistic examples.

1. DRUGS PRODUCING CHANGES IN THE CRYSTALLINE LENS

Deposits in or on the crystalline lens, in themselves may or may not be a cause for concern and thus discontinuation of the drug therapy. However, some of the drugs that can produce dramatic effects on the crystalline lens can also affect the retina and thus visual fields; therefore the initial appearance of lens changes could be considered as a possible indicator that more posterior changes could occur. Lens changes, in themselves, are unlikely to be a reason for discontinuing a medication.

(**a**) leading to the progressive development of <u>anterior</u> lens deposits. The deposits can be subjectively graded (1+ to 4 +) and visual acuity (VA) is not usually affected until a grade 3+ or 4+ is reached. Drugs reported to cause <u>anterior lens deposits</u> include phenothiazines (e.g. chlorpromazine, PoM **Largactil**[R]), and amiodarone (PoM **Cordarone-X**[R]).

(**b**) leading to the development of development of <u>posterior lens deposits /</u> <u>cataracts</u> (PSCC). Such drugs include all oral corticosteroids (e.g. hydrocortisone, PoM **Hydrocortistab**[R]; or oral prednisolone, PoM **Deltacortril**[R]), and there is increasing concern that the same ADR can develop after intensive use of nasal / tracheo-bronchial corticosteroids as well (e.g. fluticasone, PoM **Flixotide**[R], and in combinations, PoM **Seretide**[R]; beclomethasone, PoM **Beclovent**[R]). The risk for PSCC development is oral > inhaled >> topical skin > topical ocular corticosteroids. However, some ocular or systemic diseases (diabetes with kidney failure, or kidney failure alone) may predispose patients to develop PSCC following use of eye drops containing corticosteroids.

(**c**) leading to the development of discrete <u>cortical</u> opacities of the crystalline lens. The current example (disputed) relates to the cholesterol-lowering drugs (the 'statins'). Most current products (e.g. fluvastatin, PoM **Lescol**[R]; simvastatin, PoM **Zocor**[R]; atorvastatin, PoM **Lipitor**[R]) do not mention this ADR but some directories carry a standardized note to the effect that "Current long term studies do not indicate an adverse effect of ___ on the human lens". However, some directories state "Periodic ophthalmic examinations are recommended" (pravastatin, PoM **Lipostat**[R]), and one product (cerivastatin, PoM **Liobay**[R]) lists "lens opacities" in the ADR's.

2. DRUGS PRODUCING AN ALTERATION IN IOP

For medication-related changes in IOP, they can be considered in terms of the site of action in the eye and this approach should assist in predicting the magnitude of a drug-induced change in IOP. In other cases, such a simple logic will not always work. However, since sustained elevations in IOP are generally considered to be detrimental to the eye, such elevations in IOP (even if small) may well be a reason for discontinuing a medication. The clinical consequences of a drug-induced change in IOP can range from simply introducing an uncertainty to routine tonometry readings, to medications precipitating such an ocular hypo- or hyper-tensive crisis that emergency attention is needed. As a working guideline, the following values for IOP can be used when considering drug-induced IOP changes: normal IOP is 15 ± 3 mm Hg (range 10 to 20mm Hg; by applanation tonometry), modest elevation in IOP is up to 30 mm Hg, large elevations in IOP are when the pressures reach 31 to 45 mm Hg and very large elevations reflect any pressures above 45 mm Hg. For ocular hypotension, any pressure below 10 mm Hg should be carefully reviewed. The upper limit that is likely to be recorded clinically is probably close to 60 mm Hg. Different instruments have different ranges of optimum reproducibility and accuracy in measuring IOP, and this should be considered when interpreting older literature on these drug-induced changes in IOP. It is also very important to consider whether the changes are self-limiting (i.e. involve a time-dependent change and then an uneventful return to normal) or whether they are progressive and or will only resolve with intervention. Any effects on IOP also depend upon age of the patient and their natural diurnal IOP cycle.

(**a**) <u>reduction of IOP</u> from normally-expected values, or from those values
existing in a glaucomatous condition (including ocular hypertension).
These drug types are blood pressure-lowering drugs or other
cardiovascular drugs. such *beta*-adrenergic blocking drugs (e.g.
propranolol, PoM **Inderal**[R]), diuretics (e.g. acetazolamide, PoM
Diamox[R]; furosemide, PoM **Lasix**[R], hydrochlorthiazide, PoM
Hydrosaluric[R]), clonidine (e.g. PoM **Catapres**[R]), methylDOPA (e.g.
PoM **Aldomet**[R]), hydralazine (e.g. PoM **Apresoline**[R]), digoxin (PoM
Lanoxin[R]), oral antidiabetic drugs such as chlorpropamide (PoM
Diabinese[R]) and alcohol.

(**b**) <u>increase in IOP</u> from normally-expected values or additive to those
values existing in a glaucomatous condition (including ocular
hypertension). The effects are generally associated with pupil dilation and
so most of these drugs are therefore contraindicated in patients with
known narrow angles or pre-existing narrow angle glaucoma. Drugs
include cholinergic blockers (atropine-like drugs) being used for stomach
or GI tract ailments, nausea, motion sickness, irritable bowel syndrome or
urinary incontinence (e.g. dicyclomine, PoM **Merbentyl**[R]; hyoscine, P /
PoM **Buscopan**[R]; P **Kwells**[R], skin patches containing hyoscine
[scopolamine], PoM **Scopoderm-TTS**[R]; oxybutynin, P/ PoM **Ditropan**[R],
PoM **Cystrin**[R] or PoM **Oxybutynin**, generic; tolterodine, PoM
Detrusitol[R]; propiverine, PoM **Detrunorm**[R]), selective cholinergic
blockers such as ipratropium (e.g Rx **Atrovent**[R], PoM **Respontin**[R], PoM
Rinatec[R]), systemic drugs that have cholinergic-blocking side effects (e.g.
disopyramide, PoM **Rythmodan**[R]; phenothiazines such as
chlorpromazine, PoM **Largactil**[R], or prochlorperazine, PoM **Stemetil**[R]),
tricyclic antidepressants (e.g. trimipramine, PoM **Surmontil**[R], or
amitriptyline, PoM **Tryptizol**[R]) and older sedating (H_1-blocking) anti-
histamines (e.g. bromopheniramine P **Dimotane**[R], chlorpheniramine, P
Piriton[R]), indirect adrenergics or indirect serotoninergics including
SNRI's (e.g. venlafaxine; PoM **Efexor**[R]), NARI's (e.g. reboxetine, PoM
Edronax[R]), NaSSA's (e.g. mirtazapine; PoM **Zispin**[R]), MAO inhibitors
(e.g. phenelzine; PoM **Nardil**[R]), RIMA's (e.g. moclobemide; PoM
Manerix[R]), SSRI's (e.g. fluoxetine, PoM **Prozac**[R]; and fluvoxamine,
PoM **Luvox**[R]) or other medicines with indirect-acting adrenergic effects
including dexamphetamine (CD **Dexedrine**[R]) and methylphenidate (CD
Ritalin[R]). The overuse (abuse) of direct-acting adrenergics as found in
dilute solutions of xylometazoline (P **Otrivin**[R] Nasal Drops) can also
precipitate angle closure. Other drugs that can raise IOP include oral
corticosteroids (e.g. hydrocortisone, PoM **Hydrocortistab**[R]; or oral
prednisolone, PoM **Deltacortril**[R]), and the same ADR may develop after
intensive use of nasal / tracheo-bronchial corticosteroids as well (e.g.
fluticasone, PoM **Flixotide**[R]; beclomethasone, PoM **Beclovent**[R]). The risk
for development of ocular hypertension (steroid glaucoma) is oral >
inhaled >> topical skin > topical ocular corticosteroids.

(**c**) Changes in IOP or changes in ocular perfusion. This is a new area of concern that recognizes the role of ocular blood perfusion in maintaining the health of the nerve head. Some glaucomatous changes result from fluctuations in IOP or the ocular perfusion pressure; e.g. normal tension (low tension, NTG) glaucoma patients. Drugs with an anti-vasospasm action (e.g. clonidine, PoM **Catapres**[R]; diltiazem, PoM **Angitil**[R], verapamil, PoM **Securon**[R], and nifedipine, PoM **Adalat**[R]) may be beneficial in some patients, yet cause visual disturbances or further deterioration in the eye of others. Specific guidelines for patients are currently unavailable.

3. DRUGS CAUSING VISUAL FIELD CHANGES

Central visual field changes are often accompanied by substantial reduction in vision, even if the apparent fundus appearance is unremarkable. Drugs that have been reported to cause visual field changes (and for which automated visual field assessments should be carried out) include cytarabine (PoM **Cytosar**[R]), vigabatrin (PoM **Sabril**[R]) and possibly gabapentin (PoM **Neurontin**[R]), oestrogen- or progesterone-like drugs (e.g. medroxyprogesterone, PoM **Depo-Provera**[R], and some older oral contraceptives), warfarin (PoM **Coumadin**[R]), amiodarone (PoM **Cordarone-X**[R]), chloroquine (PoM **Avloclor**[R], PoM **Nivaquine**[R]), hydroxychloroquine PoM **Plaquenil**[R]), quinine (PoM **Quinine** [R]), isoniazid (PoM **Isoniazid**[R]), ethambutol (PoM **Ethambutol**[R]) and barbiturates.

4. DRUGS CAUSING COLOR VISION / PERCEPTION CHANGES

Red-green (R-G) defects have been reported following use of desferrioxamine (PoM **Desferal**[R]), isoniazid (PoM **Isoniazid**[R]), ethambutol (PoM **Ethambutol**[R]), nalidixic acid (PoM **Negram**[R]) and chloramphenicol (when used systemically). Blue-yellow (B-Y) have been reported following use of hydrochlorthiazide (PoM **Hydrosaluric**[R]), digoxin (PoM **Lanoxin**[R]), chlorpromazine (PoM **Largactil**[R]), thioridazine (PoM **Thioridazine**[R]), carbamazepine (PoM **Tegretol**[R]), phenytoin (PoM **Epanutin**[R]), vigabatrin (PoM **Sabril**[R]), chloroquine (PoM **Avloclor**[R], PoM **Nivaquine**[R]) hydroxychloroquine (PoM **Plaquenil**[R]), tranexamic acid (PoM **Cyklokapron**[R], disputed) and barbiturates. Some dramatic short-term changes in colour perception (e.g. yellow flashes ? or bluish tinges ?) can occur when there is an acute alteration in blood perfusion to the retina. Such transient changes (e.g. as originally reported for sildenafil, PoM **Viagra**[R]) need to distinguished from toxic effects. In the UK, on its release, sildenafil was not recommended for use in patients with "hereditary degenerate retinal disorders" and, logically, perhaps the same limitation should apply to all other drugs capable of causing colour vision changes ?.

5. DRUGS CAUSING CHANGES IN THE FUNDUS APPEARANCE

For most of the drugs that can affect the appearance of the fundus, patient monitoring (by periodic eye examinations by general medical practitioners, optometrists, hospital staff or ophthalmologists) is recommended by the drug companies and these recommendations should be adhered too as closely as practically possible. A family physician may request that such an eye examination be performed. The monitoring is to watch for possible early signs of a toxic reaction and could be unrewarding in the sense that little often happens from visit to visit. As recommended in the pharmaceutical directories, such patients should receive regular eye examinations and so can be sent for either a routine required eye examination (prior to starting therapy) or for a special one if symptoms are reported.

Various types of <u>disc</u> (optic nerve head) changes (e.g. some type of papilledema or papillitis) have been reported following use of isoniazid (PoM **Isoniazid**[R]), ethambutol (PoM **Ethambutol**[R]), nalidixic acid (PoM **Negram**[R]) and chloramphenicol (when used systemically), barbiturates, amiodarone (PoM **Cordarone**[R]), hydrocortisone (PoM **Hydrocortistab**[R]), prednisolone (PoM **Deltacortril**[R]), chlorpromazine (PoM **Largactil**[R]), and thioridazine (PoM **Thioridazine**[R]). <u>Macular changes</u> (oedema or pigmentary changes) have been reported following use of nalidixic acid (PoM **Negram**[R]), chloroquine (PoM **Avloclor**[R], PoM **Nivaquine**[R]), hydroxychloroquine (PoM **Plaquenil**[R]), tranexamic acid (PoM **Cyklokapron**[R], disputed), tamoxifen (PoM **Tamofen**[R]), cytarabine (PoM **Cytosar**[R]), indomethacin (PoM **Indocid**[R]) and barbiturates. <u>Paramacular disturbances</u> ("macular star", a para-macular ring or other exudates that are radially or circularly distributed around the macula) have been reported following use of indomethacin (PoM **Indocid**[R]), tamoxifen (PoM **Tamofen**[R]), or ergot alkaloids (PoM **Lingraine**[R]). Para-macular or general retinal pigment disturbances have been reported after use of indomethacin (PoM **Indocid**[R]), phenylbutazone (PoM **Butacote**[R]), chlorpromazine (PoM **Largactil**[R]), thioridazine (PoM **Thioridazine**[R]), carbamazepine (PoM **Tegretol**[R]), desferrioxamine (PoM **Desferal**[R]), chloroquine (PoM **Avloclor**[R], PoM **Nivaquine**[R]), and barbiturates.

Any of the changes in the nerve head, the macular region, the vasculature around either structure and the possible pigmentary changes that develop, may or may not be accompanied by haemorrhages. These may be discrete or gross, and may be single events or episodic. The haemorrhages may be precipitated indirectly as a result of drug-induced haemolysis or blood clots.

A summary of the types of changes reported for the posterior segment is provided overleaf -

SUMMARY OF POSSIBLE ADVERSE DRUG EFFECTS
ON THE POSTERIOR SEGMENT OF THE EYE

TYPE OF EFFECT	drugs
cataracts	chlorpromazine, amiodarone, hydrocortisone, prednisolone, fluticasone, beclomethasone, cerivastatin (?)
ocular hypotension	propranolol, acetazolamide, furosemide, hydrochlorthiazide, clonidine, methyldopa, hydralazine, digoxin, chlorpropamide, alcohol
ocular hypertension	dicyclomine, hyoscine [scopolamine], oxybutynin, ipratropium, disopyramide, chlorpromazine, prochlorperazine, trimipramine, amitriptyline, brompheniramine, chlorpheniramine, venlafaxine, reboxetine, mirtazapine, phenelzine, moclobemide, fluoxetine, fluvoxamine, dexamphetamine, methylphenidate, xylometazoline, hydrocortisone, prednisolone, fluticasone, beclomethasone
changes in ocular perfusion	clonidine, verapamil, diltiazem, nifedipine
visual field changes	cytarabine, vigabatrin, gabapentin, medroxyprogesterone, oral contraceptives (?), warfarin, amiodarone, chloroquine, hydroxychloroquine, quinine, isoniazid, ethambutol
color vision changes	desferrioxamine, isoniazid, ethambutol, nalidixic acid, chloramphenicol, hydrochlorthiazide, digoxin, chlorpromazine, thioridazine, carmamazepine, phenytoin, vigabatrin, chloroquine, hydroxychloroquine, tranexamic acid (?), sildenafil (?)
optic neuritis	isoniazid, ethambutol, nalidixic acid, chloramphenicol, amiodarone, hydrocortisone, prednisolone, chlorpromazine, thioridazine,
maculopathy	nalidixic acid, chloroquine, hydroxychloroquine, tranexamic acid (?)
perimacular disturbances	indomethacin, tamoxifen, ergot alkaloids
general RPE disturbances	indomethacin, phenylbutazone, chlorpromazine, thioridazine, carbamazepine, desferrioxamine, chloroquine

NOTE. The drugs listed in the above table are representative examples. A MIMS or BNF should be consulted for other drugs in the same classes. A more extensive coverage of this topic can be found in "**General Pharmacology for Primary Eye Care**"(Doughty) where these side effects are discussed within the fuller context of both the mechanisms and the clinical uses of the drugs. Extensive listings of drugs that might cause toxic effects to the posterior segment of the eye can be found by consulting "Drug-Induced Ocular Side Effects", 4th Edn (F.T. Fraunfelder).

MEDICAL MANAGEMENT OF GLAUCOMA.

Purpose of chapter. Chronic glaucoma (i.e. usually open-angle glaucoma) can be managed with drugs; this is the medical management as opposed to surgical management of glaucoma. This chapter will outline the different medical strategies that an ophthalmologist will try, the reasons why different medications need to be used, and what the use of any of these anti-glaucoma medications mean to glaucoma patients in terms of life-style. Such knowledge is important to facilitate effective monitoring of these therapies as part of shared-care of glaucoma patients.

The medical management of open-angle glaucoma is not a lightly-undertaken activity for, once started, the therapies generally need to be continued. Some physicians strongly support surgical intervention as the only hope for long-term prognosis, while others equally noisily argue that there is proof that medications will at least slow the rate of visual field loss associated with advancing glaucoma. Ocular hypertension (OHT) is generally equated with periodic elevations in IOP (e.g. to a daily average pressure of 25 mm Hg with a range of $\pm$ 5 mm Hg); such eyes are at risk for developing glaucomatous changes. For these and "normal tension" glaucomas (NTG), medical therapy is still largely directed towards keeping daily average IOP's closer to 18 mm Hg than 25 mm Hg (for example).

Before a decision is made to use medications to manage open-angle glaucoma, several factors need to be considered before starting the medications. The availability of full eye examination beyond fundus assessment and tonometry is important, with (if at all possible) at least some ideas of the magnitude of the diurnal changes in IOP are needed as well as when peak IOP occurs. Secondly, automated perimetry (or a chosen equivalent) should have been performed on at least 3 independent visits separated by 1 to 2 months to confirm the visual field changes. The fundus appearance (disc changes etc) and the visual field changes should be consistent. A glaucoma suspect can thus expect to make several visits to the specialist (ophthalmologist) before medications are prescribed. When medications are prescribed, the following points are very important -

(**i**) *systemic adverse drug reactions*. (**ADR**'s) The repeated use of eye drops for glaucoma can have substantial adverse reactions on autonomic function. A detailed knowledge of a patients' medications is essential for prescribing "anti-glaucoma" drugs. Such ADR's may only become apparent during the routine monitoring of a glaucoma patient on medications.

(**ii**) *concurrent systemic disease*. All patients with airways disease or cardiovascular disease should be carefully reviewed. It should be noted that patients with long standing diseases such as diabetes or high blood pressure are both less likely to show predictable responses to their anti-glaucoma medications, and more likely to show adverse drug reactions.

(iii) *gender considerations*. Open-angle glaucoma affects men and women about equally, although the IOP peaks may be higher in post-menopausal women compared to equivalent-aged men. There is no clear evidence that anti-glaucoma medications have different efficacy in men versus women, but the medication profiles of men versus women may mean that there can be differences in efficacy of the glaucoma medications.

(iv) *ethnic differences*. Ethnic groups with very darkly pigmented eyes tend to be affected with open-angle glaucoma more often. Since the efficacy of all topical anti-glaucoma drugs is often less in these groups, they are more likely to need multiple medications or concurrent systemic medications.

(v) *monitoring*. The goal of monitoring glaucoma patients on medications is to ensure freedom from ADR's, as well as to limit the chance of (rapid) deterioration in the visual fields. Patients need to be instructed on the importance of taking every dose. Reminders and encouragements may be needed at regular intervals. Many months or years are generally required before definite improvements in the visual field can be expected, any many patients will not show actual improvement.

STRATEGIES IN MEDICAL MANAGEMENT OF GLAUCOMA

There are essentially six current medical strategies that can be adopted, with many combinations also possible.

(I) *Use of beta-adrenergic blocking drugs for glaucoma*

These are the most popular current therapies for open-angle glaucoma since the visual and systemic side effects are generally minimal (compared to other anti-glaucoma medications) providing that care is taken NOT to use these drugs on the wrong patients; patient selection is thus very important for this goal to be realised !. (C/I) Contraindications for use of all topical *beta*-adrenergic blockers for glaucoma include a history of bronchospasm, bronchial asthma or any chronic airways disease or pulmonary obstruction. All of these ophthalmic *beta*-blockers are also contraindicated in patients with sinus bradycardia or any serious cardiac conduction-block, as well as patients with recent history of congestive heart failure, severe shock or trauma. (INT) Warnings for the use of topical *beta*-adrenergic blockers for glaucoma note that all of these ophthalmic *beta*-blockers should be used with caution (and perhaps not at all) if reasonable alternatives are available in patients with labile diabetes, patients who are pregnant or who are taking certain medications for high blood pressure and angina (e.g. calcium blockers such as verapamil), or vasodilators for high blood pressure (e.g. guanethidine, reserpine and clonidine). For patients with mild airway disease, a cardio-selective topical ophthalmic *beta*-blocker (betaxolol) may be used, but still at some risk of precipitating severe adverse reactions. Special Precautions (S/P) for the use of topical *beta*-adrenergic blockers for glaucoma note that all of these ophthalmic *beta*-blockers should be used cautiously, or avoided, if a patient is being medicated with systemic *beta*-blockers (for high blood pressure, arrhythmias or migraine). For any patient with blood pressure problems, monitoring pulse rate and blood pressure should be a constituent part of every eye examination.

Ophthalmic *beta*-blockers are generally for use on patients whose daily average IOP is significantly less than 30 mm Hg, i.e. closer to 25 mm Hg.

Five *beta*-adrenergic blockers drugs for ophthalmic use are currently marketed in the UK, although one is reserved for special cases only. Systemic (oral) *beta*-adrenergic blocking drugs are not used for management of glaucoma, although concurrent oral medication with these drugs could have substantial effects on the control of IOP by ophthalmic *beta*-blockers. The mechanism of action of the ophthalmic *beta*-blockers primarily involves a reduction in the net rate of aqueous humour secretion with little effect on outflow facility or the pupil. The current ophthalmic *beta*-adrenergic blocker drugs used for glaucoma therapy in the UK and their commercial products are listed below.

(**a**) timolol. This is used at the 0.25 % and 0.5 % concentration as eyedrops. This is a non-selective *beta*-adrenergic blocker with a high potential for causing broncho-pulmonary adverse effects. Products available are PoM **Timoptol**[R] and PoM **Glau-Opt**[R] (both in 5 mL bottles); unit-dose and preservative-free **Timoptol**[R] is also available. Several generic timolol 0.25 and 0.5 % eye drops (i.e. PoM **Timolol**[R] eye drops) are now marketed, but the supply of some needs to be checked (e.g. PoM **Glaucol**[R], 5 ml bottles). A special timolol viscous eye drop with gellan gum (PoM **Timoptol-LA**[R], 2.5 mL special bottles) for sustained action is also available.

(**b**) levobunolol. This is used at the 0.5 % concentration available as eyedrops in PoM **Betagan**[R] (5 mL bottles and unit-dose preparations); the 0.25 % concentration can be used but commercial products are not marketed in the UK. Generic levobunolol 0.5 % eye drops are now also available. Levobunolol is a non-selective *beta*-adrenergic blocker with a high potential for causing broncho-pulmonary adverse effects. **Betagan**[R] contains bisulphites, which can precipitate substantial allergic reactions.

(**c**) carteolol. This is used at the 1% or 2 % concentration and is available as PoM **Teoptic**[R] (5 mL bottles). Carteolol is a non-selective *beta*-adrenergic blocker with the potential for causing broncho-pulmonary adverse effects. However, as a result of its chemical structure, carteolol has some *beta*-adrenergic agonist effects (referred to as "intrinsic sympathomimetic activity", ISA) to offset some of the systemic blocking effects, and thus may also slightly improve outflow facility.

(**d**) betaxolol. This is used as a special microfine 0.25 % suspension (PoM **Betoptic**[R] **Suspension**, 5 mL bottle); an older 0.5% eye drops (PoM **Betoptic**[R],5 mL bottle) is still available. Betaxolol is a cardio-selective *beta*-adrenergic blocker introduced as the drug to overcome the limitations in the use of timolol and levobunolol. As a *beta*$_1$-selective blocker, it should not have broncho-pulmonary effects, and the special ophthalmic delivery system (microfine suspension) is designed to enhance ophthalmic absorption so that a lower concentration of drug can be used. Notwithstanding, the repeated use of betaxolol 0.5 % eye drops has still found to cause life-threatening bronchospasm in some asthmatic patients. The CSM thus advises careful monitoring, and that it should only be used in patients with airways disease if other medical options are not available.

(**e**) metipranolol. This has been used at the 0.1 %, 0.3 % and 0.6 % concentrations but is currently available, for special cases only, at the 0.1 % and 0.3 % concentrations (as PoM **Minims**[R] **Metipranolol**, unit-dose). This is a non-selective *beta*-adrenergic blocker with a high potential for causing broncho-pulmonary adverse effects. Its availability is limited because of a risk of the drug causing granulomatous or non-granulomatous uveitis; the 0.6 % concentration product was withdrawn from the UK because of case reports of this highly unusual iatrogenic disease and the same ADR has been reported for the 0.3 % solution.. Metipranolol use is restricted to patients who cannot tolerate preservative-containing ophthalmic *beta*-blockers (although unit-dose timolol is available, and so is unlikely to be used. Past experience has highlighted concerns about this type of inflammatory side effect. An orally-administered *beta*-blocker, practolol (used for high blood pressure), was withdrawn from sale in the early 1980's because the occurrence of a very severe inflammatory response (usually referred to as an oculo-muco-cutaneous syndrome).

Typical dosing and patient management schedules are variable but these drugs should <u>never</u> be used more than twice-a-day (*b.d.*) on a chronic basis. Starting doses and regimens can be with lower concentrations (i.e. 0.25 % for timolol, 1 % for carteolol; both *b.d.* dosing) and just once-a-day (timolol 0.25 % only). If a once-daily regimen is all that is wanted, some have strongly advocated that levobunolol (0.5 %) should be the drug of choice. In any of these cases, dosage increase can be achieved by prescribing the same low concentrations of timolol (0.25 %) *b.d.* instead of *o.d.* Similarly, higher dosing with can be achieved by then prescribing the higher concentration of drops (i.e. 0.5 % for timolol, levobunolol and betaxolol; 2 % for carteolol) *b.d.* Metipranolol could be used *b.d.*, with the option of two different concentrations (0.1 and 0.3 %). In most cases, providing systemic effects do not develop, *long-term ocular tolerance* is good and the patient can be maintained on the *beta*-blocker therapy (at the appropriate dose and regimen) for at least one and maybe two years without need for change.

After being started on ophthalmic *beta*-blockers, glaucoma patients will generally be seen at 2 weeks and 1 month to ensure that the desired IOP reduction has been achieved. For most patients, the prescribed therapy (if adequate) will produce the required lowering of IOP within a week (with *o.d.* or *b.d.* dosing), but some patients fail to show an adequate response and need early dosage adjustment. These initial visits are also very important to identify any systemic side effects.

Longer term follow-up / check-up generally requires visits every 2 or 3 months during the first year of therapy, with new pharmaceutical prescriptions being written at each visit. Visits after this time period need to be regularly spaced, but are dependent on individual patient responses to the medication (providing there are no marked changes in acuity, fields etc., and no adverse reactions to the medication).

Supplementing beta-blocker therapy. For some patients even maximum therapy with ophthalmic *beta*-blockers will not be adequate, while some patients can become refractory to ophthalmic *beta*-blocker therapy rather quickly (sometimes referred to as "escape" phenomena). Various supplemental options are available that could include the addition of adrenergic eye drops, the addition of miotic eye drops, topical or oral carbonic anhydrase inhibitors (see below).

Ophthalmic *beta*-blockers are currently the widest prescribed starting therapy for open angle glaucoma. However, only some patients can be treated with ophthalmic beta-blockers since the use of these ophthalmic *beta*-blockers is contraindicated in certain conditions (especially severe airways or cardiac disease). Alternatively, there may be a concern that the patient is at risk for, or has developed other side effects such as depression, loss of libido etc., or patients have developed a local intolerance to the beta-blocker eye drops (causing unacceptable eye irritation etc.). In all these types of cases, a patient has to be started on other medications.

(**II**) *Adrenergic, or adrenergic neurone blocker therapy for glaucoma*

Prior to the introduction of ophthalmic *beta*-blockers in the 1970's, adrenaline eye drops, or the use of various miotics was commonplace. Five main "adrenergic" options are currently available for management of glaucoma in the UK. These drugs have a mechanism that includes both increasing the facility of outflow (through alterations in the permeability of the vasculature adjacent to the Canal of Schlemn) as well as reducing the overall rate of secretion of aqueous humour.

Many years of clinical use of epinephrine (adrenaline) eye drops on a *b.d.s* or *t.d.s* basis has established that such adrenergic therapy is "safer" than ophthalmic *beta*-adrenergic blockers. Cases of systemic adrenergic responses to these eye drops being extraordinarily rare, but there are some limits to the use of adrenergics use, especially with current guidelines. **(S/P)** The potential for sympathomimetic effects cannot be ignored (*cf.* phenylephrine eye drops) and so the use of these drugs should be limited in patients with severe cardiovascular disease, stroke and severe peripheral circulatory problems (e.g Raynaud's syndrome), and to include the use of medications for the same conditions such as digoxin, and "sympathomimetic antagonists" (e.g. CNS *alpha*$_2$ agonists such as clonidine, drugs such as guanethidine, prazosin etc) Similarly, for any adrenergic glaucoma therapy, concurrent medication with any systemic sympathomimetics is not recommended, and should be limited or avoided in patients medicated with MAO inhibitors and any other "antidepressants affecting noradrenergic transmission", i.e. RIMA's, NARI's, NaSSA's, SNRI's etc.

(i) brimonidine 0.2 % eye drops were introduced in the UK (PoM **Alphagan**^{R}) in 1997 as a modern replacement for epinephrine (adrenaline) eye drops (see below); brimonidine eyedrops are for *b.d.s.* usage. The outflow facility is the site of a unique set of *alpha*$_2$ adrenergic receptors that are stimulated by special adrenergic agonists such as brimonidine, which also reduces aqueous secretion. Brimonidine is considered to have a lesser potential for irritating the conjunctiva (*cf.* epinephrine), but follicular conjunctivitis can still develop. **(C/I)** Known allergy to the drug or any other ingredients of the pharmaceutical; brimonidine ophthalmic solutions contain bisulphites. As a new medication, any ADR's should be reported to the CSM.

(iii) dipivefrin. Dipivefrin is dipivalyl epinephrine, i.e. the dipivalyl ester of epinephrine (adrenaline); it a pro-drug and is rapidly hydrolyzed to epinephrine by the cornea. The derivatisation improves corneal permeability by a factor of 20. Eye drops containing 0.1 % dipivefrin were introduced in the early 1980's (PoM **Propine**^{R}, 5 mL or 10 mL bottles); generic dipivefrin (5 mL bottles) were introduced in 1997 but their availability has been inconsistent, although a PoM **Dipivefrine**^{R} product is currently listed (5 mL and 10 mL bottles). Unit-dose preparations are not available. As with epinephrine, dipivefrin is generally considered as a much "safer" drug to the ophthalmic *beta*-blockers. As the prodrug of epinephrine, it only needs to be used at low doses to lower IOP effectively. **(C/I)** Known allergy to the drug or any other ingredients of the pharmaceutical; dipivefrin ophthalmic solutions contain bisulphites which can cause allergic reactions. **(C/I) (S/P)** Dipivefrin can cause mydriasis so the drug is contraindicated in patients with narrow angles and should be used with caution until the true nature of the glaucoma has been firmly established.

Dipivefrin 0.1 % is generally for *b.d.* use (not *q.d.* and is rarely used *t.d.s*) and generally for patients with average IOP's of less than 30 mm Hg. Modest reductions in IOP (i.e. 10 to 15 %) can be expected within a week and perhaps slightly greater increases over several weeks i.e up to 20 % reductions in IOP. Patient follow-up is generally as for those receiving therapy with epinephrine eye drops. If IOP control is inadequate, the therapy can be supplemented by keeping patient on dipivefrin *b.d* and adding pilocarpine eye drops at an appropriate concentration *b.d.s.* or *t.d.s.*; the dipivefrin eye drops should be instilled 10 minutes after the pilocarpine. The starting pilocarpine concentration can usually be low (e.g. 1 % or 2 % and later there is then the option to increase the pilocarpine concentration in the drops to 3 %, or 4 %). Alternatively, the dipivefrin eye drops can be maintained *b.d.*s., and topical or oral carbonic anhydrase inhibitors added.

(**iv**) epinephrine (adrenaline) eye drops. It is still available as PoM **Simplene**[R] (7.5 mL bottle, 0.5 % and 1 % eyedrops), and PoM **Eppy**[R] (7.5 mL bottles, 1 % eyedrops). (**C/I**) Known allergy to the drug or any other ingredients of the pharmaceutical. (**C/I**) (**S/P**) Adrenaline eyedrops (unlike *beta*-blocker eyedrops) can cause slight mydriasis, so are contraindicated in patients with narrow angles. Epinephrine eye drops should thus be used with caution until the nature of the glaucoma has been established. (**S/P**) The use of epinephrine eye drops should be limited or avoided in patients medicated with other sympathomimetics (e.g. MAO inhibitors, RIMA's, NARI's, SNRI's); in such patients, the systemic absorption of the eye drops may be enough to put the patient at risk for a systemic sympathetic effect.

Epinephrine eye drops will generally be used on patients with IOP's below 30 mm Hg, and are generally used *b.d.*, and perhaps even *t.d.s.*(as opposed to *o.d.*). Moderate reductions in IOP (i.e. 15 to 20 %) can be expected within a week and perhaps slightly greater increases over several weeks, i.e. up to 30 % reductions in IOP. Patient follow-up generally needs to be less rigorous compared to patients placed on ophthalmic *beta*-blockers, but visits at 1 and 3 months and then every 3 to 6 months is not unusual. The minimum of the 6 monthly check is to assess for possible irritative reactions to the conjunctiva and so is important. (**ADR**) The overall chance of development of local ocular side effects (irritation, lacrimation, rebound hyperaemia etc.) is fairly high but the chronic use of epinephrine eye drops is also notorious for causing ocular "melanosis" (also referred to as "*adrenochrome*" deposits, or adrenomelanoses). The deposits, in this drug-induced "melanosis", can be black or very dark brown and appear on the conjunctiva, within the conjunctival crypts and lacrimal gland ducts etc, and can look like mascara in early stages. The black deposit is the result of the photooxidation of epinephrine, can be irritating, and can also discolor soft contact lenses (thus the "contraindication" for using these eye drops with soft lenses). The risks of melanosis limits current use of epinephrine eye drops, although therapy does not need to be changed if it develops. Epinephrine therapy can be supplemented with pilocarpine eye drops (e.g. 1 % or 2 %, with the adrenergic being instilled 10 minutes after the miotic) or topical or oral carbonic anhydrase inhibitors could be added.

(**iv**) apraclonidine. Initially introduced as special unit-dose formulations (PoM **Iopidine**[R]) to be used as part of the surgical procedure and immediately thereafter, but now also available as a 0.5 % solution (also PoM **Iopidine**[R]) for *b.d.* use in open-angle glaucoma patients awaiting surgery. Its original indication was to ocular hypertension developing after laser surgery to the eye but it is also now approved for special cases of open-angle glaucoma. (**S/P**) Clonidine is widely used as a high blood pressure medication so apraclonidine, as a derivative of clonidine, should be used cautiously in patients with severe cardiovascular disease or severe hypertension. In addition, since the drug is potent, the risk of excess ocular or systemic hypotension must be considered. The effects of apraclonidine may be additive to any patient's anti-hypertensive medications, or any medications with sympathomimetic effects. Apraclonidine eye drops are not recommended for use with topical ophthalmic *beta*-blockers.

(**v**) guanethidine plus adrenaline. Guanethidine plus adrenaline (epinephrine) is available as PoM **Ganda**[R] Eyedrops (7.5 mL bottles), principally now for patients already established on this therapy. Two combinations are available known as "1 + 0.2" (which is guanethidine 1 % with adrenaline 0.2 %) and "3 + 0.5" (which is guanethidine 3 % with adrenaline 0.5 %). Guanethidine is an adrenergic neurone blocker that initially produces a mild adrenergic effects followed by adrenergic blocking effects (after several days of use) as a result of depleting the sympathetic neurones of adrenaline. As a result it may initially cause a slight mydriasis and little effect on IOP, but then a slight miosis and reductions in IOP of a similar magnitude to adrenaline 1 % alone. As this indirect pre-synaptic blockade develops, the post-synaptic terminals develop what is called a "supersensitivity" so if adrenaline eye drops are also used, much lower concentrations of epinephrine are needed to produce a a lowering of IOP; this is a synergistic pharmacological effect.

PoM **Ganda**[R] is generally intended for *b.d.* use, but can be used *t.d.s.* Ocular hypotensive effects of a similar or slightly larger magnitude to the use of epinephrine 1 % can be expected. As with other epinephrine-containing eye drops, patients generally need check-up visits at one month and then every 3 to 6 months. (**C/I**) Known allergy to the drug or any other ingredients of the pharmaceutical. (**S/P**) Concurrent medication with any systemic sympathomimetics is not recommended, especially with the "3 + 0.5" formulation, and should be limited or avoided in patients medicated with MAO inhibitors, NARI's, SNRI's etc, and systemic medications containing guanethidine The potential for an initial mydriasis should not be overlooked and the pharmaceutical should only be used on clearly identified cases of open angle glaucoma. The long-term adrenergic blocking effects of the combination mean that the incidence of ocular discomfort (due to conjunctival vasodilatation) after the long-term use of these eye drops is not uncommon.

(III) *Topical carbonic anhydrase inhibitors for glaucoma therapy*

Dorzolamide is a topical carbonic anhydrase inhibitor (topical CAI) for management of open angle glaucoma. Dorzolamide 2 % (PoM **Trusopt**[R]; 5 mL bottle) is indicated (UK) for management of open angle glaucoma unresponsive to *beta*-blockers, for patients for whom *beta*-blocker therapy is contraindicated or as an adjunct therapy to *beta*-blockers. A combination product of dorzolamide 2 % with timolol 0.5 % (PoM **Cosopt**[R], 5 mL bottle) is now also marketed. Dorzolamide eye drops are currently indicated for *t.d.s.* use, but can be used *b.d.* as a supplementary therapy to *beta*-blockers, adrenergics or miotics; **Cosopt**[R] is indicated for *b.d.s.* use only. (C/I) Dorzolamide eye drop use is contraindicated in patients with severe kidney diseases of any type. (S/P) Dorzolamide-containing eye drops should be used cautiously in patients with known sulphonamide drug allergy or with severe hepatic disease, although topical CAI's are not expected to produce substantial adverse systemic reactions of the type that limit the use of topical ocular *beta*-blockers (see above) or oral CAI's (see below). It remains to be seen however whether this ideal is realised in general clinical use. As new medications, all ADR's should be reported to the CSM.

(IV) *Topical prostaglandin analogue therapy for glaucoma*

Latanoprost eye drops (PoM **Xalatan**[R], 0.005 % eye drops, 2.5 mL special bottle) are indicated for management of uncomplicated open angle glaucoma where other treatments have failed or are not tolerated. This is a a prostaglandin pro-drug, specifically an ester of prostaglandin F_{2alpha}, indicated for just *o.d.* use (preferably evening), to provide equivalent hypotensive effects to timolol 0.5 %, *b.d.s.* Latanoprost appears to reduce IOP primarily by increasing the uveo-scleral outflow and so some consider that it should not be used concurrently use with miotics. Adjunct therapy with *beta*-blockers, dipivefrin, topical or oral CAI's appear to be effective and acceptable (providing there are no contraindications to such combinations). (S/P) Due to the development of severe adverse reactions, latanoprost is not indicated for use in any form of 'glaucoma' in pseudo-phakic patients or those with any other inflammatory or neovascular ocular disease. Patients on latanoprost therapy should also be carefully monitored for conjunctival (substantial hyperaemia) or iris (drug-associated heterochromia) ADR's. While the conjunctival vasodilatation and resultant irritation is an expected effect of a prostaglandin (and it unlikely to be any worse than that which can develop following chronic use of miotic; see below), the drug-related darkening of the iris pigment was unexpected (and is presumed due to recruitment of melanocytes rather then being an 'adrenochrome'-like effect, see epinephrine) . There is also come current concern that the chronic use of latanoprost eye drops could also produce darker and longer eyelashes (and even growth of a second row of eyelashes). As a new medication, any ADR's should be reported to the CSM.

(V) *Miotic therapy for glaucoma*

Miotic therapies formed the mainstay of glaucoma therapy for over 50 years, but is now only used as a starting medication on patients with average IOP's over 30 mm, or those who have very darkly pigmented eyes. While the efficacy of miotics such as pilocarpine is very much related to ocular pigmentation, concentrations of the drug are available that allow one to largely overcome the pigmentation effects, e.g. pilocarpine 4 % is usually available and concentrations as high as 10 % could be prepared by a hospital pharmacy. Lower concentrations of pilocarpine (0.5 to 2 %) are generally for use as supplements to *beta*-blocker or adrenergic therapies rather than for use as primary treatments. The miotic therapy primarily produces a reduction in IOP by increasing outflow facility, but there is some evidence that the direct-acting cholinergics can also reduce aqueous humour secretion slightly. The miosis-related increase in outflow facility can be likened to a stretching effect on the trabecular meshwork that promotes the access of the aqueous humour to the Canal of Schlemn.

(**C/I**) Repeated use of miotics as long term glaucoma therapy is to be avoided in any patient with a history of intraocular inflammation since the miotic will tend for further dilate the blood vessels in the inflamed tissue and put the patient at risk for *iris bombe*. (**S/P**) Miotic therapy is generally not indicated for use in patients with lighter pigmented (blue) eyes because of the pronounced miosis that can accompany the hypotensive action of these drugs in lightly-pigmented eyes. The repeated use of pilocarpine (or other miotics) can lead to substantial visual acuity changes (due to pseudomyopia) in younger glaucoma patients. Pronounced ciliary body spasm that may also accompany the initial use of these drugs, but an adaptive effect is usually seen within a week or so. (**ADR**) miotic therapy tends to be uncomfortable, and cosmetically unappealing (due to cholinergic vasodilatation on the bulbar conjunctiva). Excessive lacrimation and even epiphora can also be present. When starting a patient on pilocarpine or other miotics, it is important to carefully select patients and provide appropriate counselling for the potential local ocular side effects. (**ADR**) (**S/P**) Currently, there is renewed debate as to whether miotic eye drops - in general - should be considered as risk for bronchospasm is either asthmatic patients or those with cardiac insufficiency (since parasympathetic effects on the lungs and heart have been reported following the use of eye drops containing indirect acting cholinergics or carbachol).

Miotics available for general use are as follows. Pilocarpine is available at the 0.5, 1, 2, 3 and 4 % concentrations as PoM **Isopto Carpine**[R] (10 mL bottles) and in a range of generic products. Pilocarpine 1, 2 and 4 % concentrations were also available as PoM **Sno-Pilo**[R] (10 mL bottles, discontinued 8/1999). A 4 % pilocarpine gel formulation (PoM **Pilogel**[R], 5 g tube) is also available. Carbachol is available at the 3 % concentration as

PoM **Isopto Carbachol**[R] (10 mL bottles), but other concentrations (e.g. 1.5 and 0.75 %) could be prepared by a major hospital pharmacy. Physostigmine is no longer commercially. Eye drops containing 0.25 or 0.5 % physostigmine or physostigmine 0.25 % with pilocarpine 2 % or 4 % could also be prepared by a hospital pharmacy. Eye drops containing echothiophate or demecarium are reserved for use for patients who are responsive to miotics (and cannot be medicated with other anti-glaucoma drugs) and who need a substantial and long-lasting effect, e.g. the addition of echothiophate *o.d* to a *q.d.s.* regimen of pilocarpine 4 %.

Miotic therapy should be initiated *t.d.s* or *q.d.s.* at a concentration or dose commensurate with the ocular hypotensive effect required (with the ultimate goal of reducing the IOP to less than 20 mm Hg). The full effect does not have to be produced immediately, i.e. a patient can be started on a lower concentration such as 2 % pilocarpine for a few weeks then shifted up to a higher concentration and / or a combination with a second miotic (e.g. physostigmine) added where appropriate, especially for overnight coverage. With the introduction of pilocarpine 4 % gel, this provides an extra option for *o.n.* use, without the need to further increase the pilocarpine concentration with special hospital preparations. Little further increases in efficacy can be expected above the 6 % concentration of pilocarpine, unless the ocular pigment is very dense. If intensive miotic therapy is still inadequate, supplementation can be with *beta*-blockers, epinephrine or dipivefrin, topical or oral carbonic anhydrase inhibitors.

As a last alternative, the pilocarpine insert (PoM **Ocusert**[R]) P-20 or P-40 may be tried especially if a patient is having difficulty with eye drop instillation, or maintaining a *q.d.s.* regimen. These medical devices deliver pilocarpine at a constant rate to the ocular surface. The P-20 stands for 20 *u*g/hr and the P-40 for 40 *u*g/ hr. The patient requires careful instruction on how to, and when to insert and remove / replace the device. The patient must be able to tolerate the insert (that can be likened to hard contact lens) as well as be sufficiently aware of it (in case it falls out). Generally, the device will be in place for 7 days before being replaced. The Ocuserts must be stored in a refrigerator

(**VI**) *Oral carbonic anhydrase inhibitors (CAI's) for glaucoma therapy*

All topical anti- glaucoma therapies (except topical CAI's) can be supplemented with oral CAI's. These drugs enter the eye (via the ciliary circulation and ciliary epithelium) to inhibit the carbonic anhydrase-dependent aqueous humour secretion.These drugs were used substantially 1950's and 1960's, but are rarely used now because "avoidable" adverse drug reactions commonly encountered. Sustained-release capsules of acetazolamide (e.g. 250 mg, PoM **Diamox**[R] **SR**) are used as an adjunct to the topical glaucoma medications; the special slow-release capsules (also known as *sequels*) should be used *o.d.* or *b.d.s.* Acetazolamide may also be used orally or *i.v.* prior to an eye operation to lower IOP. Another carbonic anhydrase inhibitor, dichlorphenamide (e.g. PoM **Daranide**[R], 50 mg *tab*), was discontinued in October, 1996 (but could still be used by a hospital).

(**S/P**) A range of general adverse effects (tiredness, malaise etc.) can develop following oral CAI therapy. As diuretics, oral CAI's can lower blood pressure and reduce blood K^+ levels hypokalaemia) so blood K^+ levels and other electrolytes data should be regularly be available, and K^+ supplements considered.(**C/I**) Oral CAI's should not be used (as general anti-glaucoma drugs) in patients severe kidney dysfunction (who will likely have electrolyte imbalances), and should also be avoided if possible in patients with adrenal insufficiencies or hepatic dysfunction. (**S/P**) Oral CAI's should be used cautiously in patients with a history kidney disease. With such considerations, the general adverse effects (tiredness, malaise etc.) should be minimised. (**INT**) Concurrent therapies of oral CAI's with high doses of certain NSAID's (e.g. acetylsalicylic acid or other salicylates) or systemic corticosteroids (e.g. prednisolone and perhaps other steroids in general) can produce severe hepatic dysfunction. For similar reasons, concurrent therapy with anti-coagulants (e.g. heparin) is also not recommended. (**ADR**) A widely publicised ADR with oral CAI's relates to a unique type of allergic or hypersensitivity reaction; in the extreme, this can cause severe rashes and / or a general blood dyscrasia. Therefore, beyond checking for allergy to carbonic anhydrase inhibitors *per se*, a check also needs to be made for potential allergy to related compounds. The carbonic anhydrase inhibitors show some chemical identity to sulphonamide anti-infective drugs (although these do not act as CAI's or have diuretic actions) and to some oral anti-diabetes drugs because these are sulphonylurea's (e.g. chlorpropamide, PoM **Diabinese**[R]). The sulphonamides may also be referred to as folic acid antagonists (because this is the mechanism of their anti-bacterial action) and the oral anti-diabetes drugs as oral hypoglycemic drugs (because they promote insulin release and thus lower the blood sugar levels). The limitation for oral anti-diabetes drugs does not apply to drugs that are not sulphonylurea's (e.g. metformin and acarbose).

SOURCES OF DRUG INFORMATION AND REGULATIONS
PERTAINING TO DRUG USE BY OPTOMETRISTS, ORTHOPTISTS
and OPTICIANS IN THE UNITED KINGDOM.

Purpose of chapter. The use of medicines is defined by law and only those
medicines designated for use by optometrists, orthoptists or opticians
should be used on the public at-large. The goal of this chapter is to review
the legalities of the availability and use of medicines, as it applies to
optometrists (ophthalmic opticians).

The use of drugs by optometrists is determined by the MEDICINES ACT.
This act was originally prepared in 1968, and was passed into law in 1972.
It was further defined for optometrists in 1978, and has several other
modifications (in 1983 and 1984) with the last being 1989. The act, and its
consequences, are periodically reviewed, especially by a drug advisory
panel (with optometrists being represented). The main result is the
preparation of the "OPTOMETRIST'S FORMULARY" by the (British) College
of Optometrists. This formulary (3rd edition published December, 1998)
defines which medicines can be legitimately used and supplied by
optometrists within their normal scope of practice. By default, the
Medicines Act defined drug use by dispensing optometrists and orthoptists
by not including them. Optometrists, orthoptists and dispensing opticians
may well be involved in the observation of and / or providing advice to their
clients on the use of GSL products or P Medicines that are generally
available to the public at-large.

The Opticians Act (as relating to optometry) states, where it appears to a
"registered optician" that a person consulting him is suffering from an injury
or disease of the eye, the "optician" shall except in an emergency or where
otherwise owing to special circumstances impracticable or inexpedient to do
so, take the prescribed steps to refer that person to a registered medical
practitioner for advice and treatment. The emergency definition is open to
responsible interpretation by optometrists in the UK, depending on patient
circumstance, when the events occur and the location of the practice.

Classification of drugs relevant to use by optometrists

The drugs covered by the MEDICINES ACT are listed later in this chapter.
Details of which drugs fall into which category under the Medicines Act can
be found in a book called the Medicines and Poisons Guide published by the
Pharmaceutical Press. Various directories are also available that allow for
the easy identification of these categories (see listing at end). The Act was
devised to make the process of drug (medicines) administration, supply and
sale as easy, safe and uncomplicated as possible. The sections of the Act
relevant to optometrists are part III, sections 51, 52, 57 and 58; orthoptists
are not included in these sections. Medicines are usually supplied by
pharmacists, unless they have a special exemption (and are General Sales

List pharmaceuticals). For all other pharmaceuticals, a primary stipulation for the access and sale of medicines for all "users" (including physicians and other health care providers) is that it should take place from registered pharmacies, and should only be by or under the supervision of a registered pharmacist. This very rigid stipulation was relaxed to allow for the professional use of drugs by optometrists. This relaxation took the form of exemptions (exceptions) by which a registered pharmacist can supply an optometrist with certain pharmaceuticals (drugs) on receipt of an official signed order, i.e. a written request on the optometrists' letterhead. These pharmaceuticals could be for diagnostic or therapeutic use. The order and the resultant sale must stipulate the exact quantities required and the receiving optometrist is thus legally responsible for keeping records on the ultimate use of these medicines. The optometrist, depending on the stipulations of the sale, is allowed to either use these pharmaceuticals (drugs) on their patients as appropriate and as part of eye evaluation, or to administer these pharmaceuticals to their patients for management of certain emergencies. Overall, these lists include some 30 drugs, although a number of these are essentially the same drug in terms of clinical use. Under special circumstances, the optometrist may supply these drugs to their patients if the drug / pharmaceutical is identified as one for which there is a "Use and Supply" designation or category. (as opposed to a "Use only" designation); this can apply to GSL, P or PoM designated products (see below) relevant to eye care. In such cases, the patients can then administer the pharmaceuticals to themselves. This latter category includes consideration of the definition of emergency measures (see later).

Classification of medicines within the Medicines Act

The Medicines Act defines medicines by placing them on one of three main lists or categories. The designation is for pharmaceuticals, not drugs *per se* since a certain drug as an ingredient in a pharmaceutical can be found in products designated under more than one category. The three categories are

(1) the General Sales List, denoted by GSL and as defined by Section 51 of the Medicines Act. Drugs listed under (G)SL are generally available for use by the public at-large. Their designation reflects that fact that the nature of the ingredients, the concentrations of the drugs and the designated use of these is such that they are considered as safe. Thus, the public can obtain these medicines without supervision and assume responsibility for using the product as directed, reading (and respecting) any warnings / precautions about the use of these medicines and to keep them away from other potential users (e.g. children !). These GSL medicines can generally be found on the shelves in a chemist or pharmacy store, or even a supermarket or corner store, i.e. these products can be directly sold to the general public. Any retailer may sell as GSL medicine providing that the sale premises are permanent and secure (by appropriate locks etc.); any optometrists office

satisfies such criteria. The GSL medicines are sometimes referred to as off-the-shelf but the term over-the-counter (OTC) is just as widely used. More recently, some eye drops and eye salves are being classified as non-medicinal and so do not have a GSL or even P designation; these include eye vitamin products. Directories are published that list these products under an OTC category. Included in such off-the-shelf products will be contact lens wear products, including saline, cleaning, disinfecting solutions, re-wetting drops, and most recently, a range of non-medicinal (cosmetic) eye drops.

(ii) Pharmacy Medicines, denoted by P (occasionally as PM) and as defined by Section 52 of the Medicines Act. This is the in between list; if a pharmaceutical is not on the GSL or PoM (see below) lists, then it is usually on the Pharmacy Medicines list. Drugs included on this list will generally be sold or supplied from a registered pharmacy under the "supervision" of a registered pharmacist, although some products will only be available from a hospital pharmacy for use by professionals (HP). The P products are can also referred to as over-the-counter (OTC) and specific directories are published that list these products under an OTC category. The P designation is simply meant to indicate that the ingredients, their concentrations and their indicated uses are such that they are generally safe for use by the public at-large without medical supervision. However, their ingredients, the concentrations and their indicated uses are such that a control step for the supply is included so that a professional can both monitor their supply and make decisions on the suitability of the patient (customer) to use these products; this control step largely relates to ensuring that certain warnings / precautions will be provided to the end-user at the time of the sale, i.e. the pharmacists will be expected to ask several specific questions relating to the listed indications, contraindications (**C/I**), specific precautions (**S/P**), possible drug-drug interactions (**INT**) and (sometimes) provide an addition warning on potential adverse drug reactions (**ADR**'s). From an ocular perspective, these P products include certain eye drops for relief of irritated eyes, artificial tears, astringents and some eyewashes. The P designation also includes a very large number of other general remedies for allergies, alimentary tract disorders, skin irritation, personal hygiene and sleep disorders. While the end-user assumes responsibility for the correct use of the product, the pharmacist or other health care professional assumes the responsibility for providing the end-user with the appropriate "instructions for use". Rather than being off-the-shelf, these products will generally be supplied by the pharmacist on receipt of a specific verbal request from a consumer. Usually only single products will be sold under such a P designation, i.e. the availability of multiple products should be via a general medical practitioner (or equivalent) or via the office of a professional. When P medicines are used in the office of a professional or supplied to a patient from such a practice, the professional also assumes the responsibility for instructing the patient on the use of the pharmaceutical.

Details of the Pharmacy Medicines for ophthalmic use can be found in several published sources (see end of chapter). Some other non-prescription products fall into the P category but will not be supplied to a member of the general public. These products, including drugs for diagnostic use, can be generally supplied in bulk to an optometrist for professional use, providing a signed order is presented to a pharmacist. The signed order simply needs to be on the optometrist's letterhead and request the "supply" of the designated pharmaceutical and the quantity required.

(iii) Prescription Only Medicines, denoted by PoM or POM and as defined by Section 58 of the Medicines Act. The term applies to several hundred different pharmaceuticals, and for the most part, the term can be taken literally, i.e. the pharmaceutical should only be available via a prescription written by a general medical practitioner, dentist or veterinarian. However, by special exemptions, optometrists may purchase a number of these prescription-only medicines for their professional use. A signed order must be presented to a pharmacist and simply needs to be on the optometrists' letterhead and be a request for the "supply" of the designated pharmaceutical and the quantity required, e.g. 36 x 5 g tubes of Atropine Eye Ointment 1 %. Some of these PoM pharmaceuticals that the optometrist has access to are of the type that could be used in an emergency (see later). Overall, the restricted access is more to ensure the safety of the general public since as a general guideline, PoM listings designate those pharmaceuticals that contain drugs (or higher concentrations of drugs) for which there should be some supervision for their use. The risks for ADR's are generally higher for PoM versus P or GSL products, with the key difference being one of the quantity of the drug in the pharmaceutical and thus the amount that might reasonably be taken as a single dose.

The classification of medicines is regularly reviewed, and pharmaceuticals that were once considered only for PoM classification are now available as Pharmacy Medicines. Such changes are likely to occur whenever it can be established that the frequent use of a pharmaceutical by the public at-large produces no significant adverse reactions or drug-drug interactions. In such cases there is no longer a good reason for keeping the PoM designation; a P Medicine may revert to PoM designation however if an unacceptably high incidence of ADR's is reported. For most new PoM designated drugs / pharmaceuticals, a specific note in the directories will be found stating that the Committee on the Safety of Medicines (CSM) must be informed if any adverse reactions are encountered.

TOPICAL OPHTHALMIC DRUGS FOR USE BY OPTOMETRISTS
Each drug is listed along with its designation of P (use and supply), PoM (use and supply) and PoM (use only). Details include those listed in the .
Optometrists Formulary, *while notes of interpretation made by the author are in italics.*

USE AND SUPPLY, i.e. the optometrist may administer pharmaceuticals containing these drugs to patients as part of their normal professional practice and also supply these pharmaceuticals to their patients on the condition that "The sale or supply shall only be in the course of their professional practice and only in an emergency"). *Optometrists may sell and supply all GSL and P Medicines relevant to their professional practice.*

Staining agents - fluorescein sodium (P), rose bengal (P). *Logically reserved for use only (because there is no patient-originating use for these).*

Mydriatics and Decongestants (sympathomimetics) - phenylephrine hydrochloride up to 10 % (P/ PoM), xylometazoline hydrochloride (P), naphazoline salts (PoM). Adrenaline (P) and ephedrine (P) salts are also listed but commercial P Medicine are not available. *Logically, supply and use of phenylephrine should be limited to P products 0.12 % only.*

Antiallergics - antazoline (up to 1 %) (P), sodium cromoglicate up to 2 % (eyedrops, P only). A 4 % ointment is listed, but is no longer available. *This category logically extends to levocabastine (P) products.*

Artificial tears, lubricants, eyewashes, moisturisers, and irrigation solutions - SL / P products - *to logically include any sterile products suitable for eye irrigation (containing saline / NaCl, witch hazel or other natural extracts, zinc sulphate) and / or containing viscosity-enhancing polymers (e.g. polyvinyl alcohol, hypromellose, hydroxyethylcellulose, dextran, povidone / polyvidone, Carbomer, hyaluronate) designated as artificial tears or ocular lubricants, moisturisers or re-wetting solutions. Also includes P products containing white or yellow or liquid paraffin, lanolin.*

Cycloplegics and mydriatics (anti-muscarinics) - atropine sulphate (PoM), cyclopentolate hydrochloride (PoM), homatropine hydrobromide (PoM), tropicamide (PoM); hyoscine hydrobromide (scopolamine, PoM) is listed but not generally marketed any longer. *Logically, atropine or homatropine could be supplied for short-term home use prior to eye examinations, but the home use of the other antimuscarinics is questionable and does not logically extend to treatment of chronic conditions.*

Antimicrobial agents - chloramphenicol eye drops (up to 0.5 %) (PoM), chloramphenicol eye ointment (up to 1%) (PoM), propamidine isethionate eye drops (P), dibromopropamidine isethionate eye ointment (P); sulphacetamide is listed (PoM; up to 30 %) but is no longer available. *Logically, the use and supply of chloramphenicol should be such that a sufficient dose of the drug is delivered to be effective, e.g. q.d.s. dosing and "continue for 48 h after clinical cure" (MIMS guidelines for use). Efficacy of propamidine salts for prophylaxis following corneal damage or minor injury has not been established.*

Miotics (parasympathomimetics) - pilocarpine salts (PoM), and carbachol (PoM); bethanecol is also listed but not available as eye drops. *Logically, any supply of miotics to a patient by an optometrist should be restricted to eye drops and only then under very special circumstances. Such use and supply does not logically extend to treatment of chronic conditions.* Two other miotics ("anticholinesterases") are also listed but neither neostigmine (PoM), or physostigmine (PoM) are available as eye drops.

USE ONLY, i.e. the optometrist may administer pharmaceuticals containing these drugs but not supply these pharmaceuticals to a patient for self-use under any circumstances, *or use them on themselves* !).

Topical anesthetics - amethocaine hydrochloride (PoM), oxybuprocaine hydrochloride (PoM), proxymetacaine hydrochloride (PoM), lignocaine hydrochloride (PoM). *This includes combinations with fluorescein.*

Antimicrobial agents - framycetin sulphate (PoM). *While use is permitted, logically this use is of questionable value since it would require a patient to return to the practice at regular intervals to receive a reasonable dose of the drug for management of an infection or a possible infection.*

Alpha adrenoceptor blocker (miotic) - thymoxamine (PoM) listed but no longer available. Anti-inflammatory agent - oxyphenbutazone ointment (PoM); listed but no longer available.

Detailed records of pharmaceuticals under the GSL or P categories do not need (according to the law) to be kept by an optometrist (although details should best be included in a patients' records). Detailed pharmacy stock and use records should be kept for all PoM designated pharmaceuticals used in the practice. In addition, when optometrists supply their patients with "exempted" PoM designated pharmaceuticals, detailed records should be kept. The optometrist may also re-label pre-packaged pharmaceuticals (preparations) without holding a manufacturers licence for assembly of pharmaceuticals; there is no requirement to do this. Pharmacy and GSL medicines should not be relabelled (unless a specific approval and licence is granted to the individual optometrist).

However, under the provisions of the regulations for labelling of a "dispensed medicinal product", such a label must state the name of the patient (who must be physically present), the directions for use, the words "Keep out of reach of children", the phrase "For external use only", the date of the supply and the name and address of the supplying optometrist.

SOURCES OF INFORMATION ON PHARMACEUTICALS

No single directory is available that lists all pharmaceuticals and also provides information on their designation for use or supply. The following sources are useful -

1. MIMS. The Monthly Index of Medical Specialities is published monthly by Haymarket Medical Ltd. It is updated every month and supplied to medical practitioners and pharmacists. It can be obtained by subscription-only from MIMS Subscription, 3-4 Hardwick St., London EC1R 4RY. The cost is just a few pounds / month. The MIMS directory contains details of all PoM preparations that are available as brand-name

pharmaceuticals but generally does not list generic preparations. The MIMS lists some P medicines that are identifiable only because of the lack of a prescription-only designation. The MIMS contains general details on the indications for use of all PoM preparations, the reasons for these indications, brief guidelines on the use and follow-up as well as designations for contraindications (C/I), special precautions (S/P), possible drug interactions (INT) and adverse drug reactions (ADR).

2. BNF. The British National Formulary is a joint publication of the British Medical Association and the Royal Pharmaceutical Society of Great Britain. It is published twice-a-year. The BNF should be available from major booksellers or from the publishers (The Pharmaceutical Press, Royal Pharmaceutical Society of Great Britain, 1 Lambeth High St., London SE1 7JN, England). The cost is a few pounds. The BNF contains details of all PoM medicines that are available as designated brand-name products (branded medicines) from pharmaceutical companies, as well as various non-proprietary (generic) formulations that are available from pharmacies (including hospital pharmacies). The BNF also includes lists of some P medicines that can be identified simply because the lack of a PoM designation. The BNF also identifies PoM pharmaceuticals which can dispensed in limited quantities as P medicines (by a pharmacist). The BNF contains limited details of the indications for use or the practical use of pharmaceuticals as well as detailed lists of potential drug-drug interactions. A useful supplement to MIMS, but since it is only updated bi-annually, it is likely to be out of date for use in clinical practice !.

3. ABPI COMPENDIUM of DATA SHEETS. This reference text (over 2000 pages) is published by Datapharm Publications Ltd (12 Whitehall, London SW1A 2DY), but copies may be difficult to obtain. Formerly called the ABPI Data Sheet Compendium, it contains information - supplied by the manufacturer's of the pharmaceuticals - on the use of the products. Each company has a section and their pharmaceuticals are sequentially listed with details of the presentation (how supplied), recommended doses, contraindications, warnings, special precautions, interactions, adverse drug reactions and overdose management. Specials details on the pharmaceutical compatibilities are provided where relevant. In many cases, the Data Sheets are similar to those in USA and Canada-based directories and provide the reasons for the S/P, INT or ADR categories found in MIMS.

4. Chemist and Druggist Guide to OTC Medicines. This annual directory is for Pharmacists and Pharmacy Assistants and is published as a supplement to the pharmacy trade magazine Chemist and Druggist. Subscriptions for Chemist and Druggist may be obtained from Benn Publications Ltd., Sovereign Way, Tonbridge, Kent TN9 1RW, but the supplement can be obtained as a separate item for just a few pounds. The supplement contains listings of many GSL and P Medicines (with the P medicines clearly identified) along with brief details of the indications for use and recommended usage. A significant number of the product listings include colour photographs of the packaging for the preparations.

5. OTC Directory. Treatments for Common Ailments. This annual directory is published by the PAGB (Promoting Responsible Consumer Health Care) and is designed to provide details of GSL (and a few P medicines) pharmaceuticals available for general use. Copies may be obtained from PAGB, Vernon House, Sicilian Avenue, London WC1 2QH. The listings are limited but do include details of the ingredients or the pharmaceuticals and essentially what is written on the packaging as "instructions for use". The directory does however provide colour illustrations of all of the packages for easy identification.

6. British Chapter of the American Academy of Optometry WWW internet site. A regularly-updated listing of current UK pharmaceuticals relevant to eye care (excluding contact lens care products) is maintained at <**http://www.academy.org.uk**>.

7. College of Optometrists "Optometrists Formulary" is published in paper / loose-leaf copy every few years; it includes listings of many current UK ophthalmic pharmaceuticals and is currently in its 3rd edition. Copies may be obtained from 42 Craven St., London WC2N 5NG.

REPORTING ADVERSE REACTIONS TO MEDICINES

Optometrists have a responsibility to report the occurrence of any adverse reaction (ADR) to their use or patient use of medicines as observed in the course of professional practice. Discussion of ocular ADR's can be made through the British Chapter of the American Academy of Optometry WWW internet site <http://www.academy.org.uk>.

Yellow Card Scheme - this card scheme, on bright yellow forms, is designed to allow for reporting on any suspected adverse reactions to ophthalmic products. These reactions include those to contact lenses, associated solutions (fluids) and other related products and medicines sold, supplied or used by the optometrist. For optometrists, these ADR's will have been observed as part of the eye examination performed by the optometrist, optician or orthoptists in their professional practice, and is thus the means by which an optometrist can also report any suspected ADR that is apparently associated with patient use of other pharmaceuticals or as the result of other forms of self-medication. The yellow card requests details of all suspected reactions, ocular, visual or ocular motor and applies to any drugs or form of drug treatment (including vaccines); the practitioner does not have to prove the association between the observed ADR and the medication use. Where appropriate, the patient's medical practitioner should be informed of the ADR, and the yellow card requires that the date that the medical practitioner was informed should be specified. The yellow card is returned to the Medical Assessor for Adverse Reactions on the Committee on Safety of Medicines (CSM). The yellow reporting form is also found in the BNF and the OTC directory. The yellow card requires the reporting of the BRAND name of the pharmaceuticals, the frequency of use of the pharmaceuticals (or contact lenses) and when the use was started and ended. The designated purpose of the use of the pharmaceuticals also needs to be provided. Details of the suspected adverse drug reactions, when they started and ended and the outcome also need to be provided. On filing information on a suspected adverse drug reaction to the CSM, the practitioner should be able to request information on equivalent reports.

Green Card Scheme for Optometrists - this report card, on darker green forms, was designed to allow for reporting on any suspected adverse reactions to any medicines (GSL, P or POM designated) to the College of Optometrists. It has now been superseded by the Yellow Card scheme (see above).

BIBLIOGRAPHY for UK edition of
Drugs, Medications and the Eye

Chapter 1 - **PRINCIPLES OF DRUG ACTION**
Doughty MJ (1991) Basic principles of pharmacology. In -
Clinical Ocular Pharmacology and Therapeutics (ed.
Onofrey B). JB Lippincott, Philadelphia. Chapter 1, pp.
1-38.

Chapter 2 - **MEDICATIONS or UNDERSTANDING A
PATIENTS MEDICATION LIST AND MAKING OFFICE
RECORDS**
Elliott DB (1997) Clinical Procedures in Primary Eye
Care. Butterworth - Heinemann, Oxford
Gibaldi M (1984) Biopharmaceutics and Clinical
Pharmacokinetics. Lea & Febiger, Philadelphia.
Mitra AK (ed) (1993) Ophthalmic Drug Delivery Systems.
Marcel Dekker Inc, New York.

Chapter 3 - **OPHTHALMIC PHARMACEUTICALS**
Burstein NL (1980) Corneal cytotoxicity of topically
applied drugs, vehicles and preservatives. Surv
Ophthalmol. 25: 15-30.
Chiambaretta F, Pouliquen P, Rigal D (1997) Allergie et
conservateurs. A propos de trois cas d'allergie au
chlorure de benzalkonium. J Fr Ophtalmol. 20: 8-16.
Christie CL, Meyler JG (1997) Contemporary contact lens
care products. Contact Lens Anterior Eye 20 (suppl):
S11-S17.
German EJ, Hurst MA, Wood D (1997) Eye drop
container delivery: a source of response variation ?.
Ophthal Physiol Opt 17: 196-204.
Ludwig A, van Haeringen NJ, Bodelier VMW, Van
Ooteghem M (1992) Relationship between precorneal
retention of viscous eyedrops and tear fluid composition.
Int Ophthalmol. 16: 23-26.
Mondino BJ, Salamon SM, Zaidman GW (1982) Allergic
and toxic reactions on soft contact lens wearers. Surv
Ophthalmol. 26: 337-344.
Mullen W, Shephered W, Labovitz J (1973) Ophthalmic
preservatives and vehicles. Surv Ophthalmol. 17: 469-
483.
Papadimitriou JT (1983) Complications of preservatives in
contact lens solutions. Austral J Optom. 66: 220-226.
Pearson FC (1990) Aseptic pharmaceutical manufacturing
Technology for the 1990's (Olson WP, Groves MJ,
eds), pp. 75-100.
Roth HW (1991) Polyquad-induced mixed solution
syndrome in contact lens wear. Contactologica 13: 8-11.
Tan B (1974) Hypersensitivity and allergic reactions to
ophthalmic drugs. Austral J Optom. 57: 14-21.
Wilson FM (1979) Adverse external ocular effects of
topical ophthalmic medications. Surv Ophthalmol. 24:
57-88.
Wilson LA (1996) To preserve or not to preserve, is that
the question ?. Br J Ophthalmol. 80: 583-584.
Wilson-Holt N, Dart JKG (1989) Thimerosal
keratoconjunctivitis, frequency, clinical spectrum and
diagnosis. Eye 3: 581-587.
Wood CA (1909) A System of Ophthalmic Therapeutics.
Cleveland Press, Chicago.

Chapter 4 - **EYEWASHES, OPHTHALMIC DYES, STAINS
and TOPICAL OCULAR ANAESTHETICS**
Topical drug delivery to the eye
Balant LP, Doelker E, Buri P (1990) Prodrugs for the
improvement of drug absorption via different routes of
administration. Eur J Drug Metab Pharmacokin. 15:
143-153.
Ellis PP, Wu P-Y, Pfoff DS et al. (1992) Effect of
nasolacrimal occlusion on timolol concentrations in the
aqueous humor of the human eye. J Pharm Sci. 81: 219-
220.
Huang TC, Lee DA (1989) Punctal occlusion and topical
medications for glaucoma. Am J Ophthalmol. 107: 151-
155.
Lahdes KK, Huupponen RK, Kaila TJ (1994) Ocular
effects and systemic absorption of cyclopentolate
eyedrops after canthal and conventional application.
Acta Ophthalmol. 72: 698-702.
Maurice DM, Mishima S (1984) Ocular Pharmacokinetics.
In - Handbook Experimental Pharmacology (Sears ML,
ed). Springer-Verlag, Berlin, pp. 19-116.
Peyman GA (1977) Antibiotic administration in the
treatment of bacterial endophthalmitis. II. Intravitreal
injections. Surv Ophthalmol. 21: 332-346.
Sanbron GE, Anand R, Torti RE et al. (1992) Sustained-
release ganciclovir therapy for treatment of
cytomegalovirus retinitis. Arch Ophthalmol. 110: 188-
195.
Sasaki H, Yamamura K, Nishida K et al. (1996) Delivery
of drugs to the eye by topical application. Prog Retinal
Eye Res. 15: 583-620.
Urtti A, Salminen L (1993) Minimizing systemic
absorption of topically administered ophthalmic drugs.
Surv Ophthalmol. 37: 435-456.
Eyewashes, lid scrubs, , hypertoncis, irrigation solutions
Clark MJ, Chapman ND, Noyelle RM, Lancaster L (1989)
An open multiple dose study of Optrex Eye Lotion in
eye irritation due to hayfever. Br J Clin Pract. 43: 357-9.
Galin MA, Davidisn R, Schacter N (1966)
Ophthalmologial use of osmotic therapy. Am J
Ophthalmol. 62: 629-634.
Key JE (1996) A comparative study of eyelid cleaning
regimens in chronic blepharitis. CLAO J 22: 209-212.
Luxenberg MN, Green K (1971) Reduction in corneal
edema with topical hypertonic agents. Am J Ophthalmol.
71: 847-853.
Marisi A, Aquavella JV (1975) Hypertonic saline solution
in corneal edema. Ann Ophthalmol (Chic). 7: 229-233.
Smith RE, Flowers CW (1995) Chronic blepharitis: A
review. CLAO J. 21: 200-207.
Ophthalmic dyes and stains
Crook TG (1979) Fluorescein as an aid in pachometry.
Am J Optom Physiol Opt. 56: 124-127.
Emran N, Sommer A (1979) Lisamine green staining in
the clinical diagnosis of xerophthalmia. Arch
Ophthalmol. 97: 2333-2335.
Feenstra RPG, Tseng SCG (1992) Comparison of
fluorescein and rose bengal staining. Ophthalmology 99:
605-617.

Gass JDM (1968) A fluorescein angiography study of macular dysfunction secondary to retinovascular diease. Arch Ophthalmol. 80: 535-617.

Hara T, Inami M, Hara T (1998) Efficacy and safety of fluorescein angiography with orally administered sodium fluorescein. Am J Ophthalmol. 126: 560-564.

Hochheimer BF (1971) Angiography of the retina with indocyanine green. Arch Ophthalmol. 86: 564-565.

Holly FJ, Lamberts DW (1979) Sorption of high molecular weight fluorescein by Polymacon hydrogel contact lenses. Intraoc Lens Contact Lens J. 5(4): 160-174.

Jalbert I, Sweeney DF, Holden BA (1999) The characteristics of corneal staining in successful daily and extended disposable contact lens wearers. Clin Exptl Optom 82: 4-10.

Justice J, Soper JW (1976) An improved method of viewing topical fluorescein. Trans Am Acad Ophthalmol Otolaryngol. 81: OP927-OP928.

Kame RT (1979) Basic considerations in fitting hydrogel lenses. J Am Optom Assoc. 50: 295-298.

Kimura SJ (1951) Fluorescein paper. A simple means of ensuring the use of sterile fluoresein. Am J Ophthalmol. 34: 446-447.

Korb DR, Herman JP (1979) Corneal staining subsequent to sequential fluorescein instillations. J Am Optom Assoc. 50: 361-367.

Kronning E (1954) Conjunctival and corneal stainability with rose bengal. Am J Ophthalmol. 38: 351-367.

Laroche RR, Campbell RC (1988) Qunatitative rose bengal staining technique for external ocular disease. Ann Ophthalmol (Chic) 20: 274-276.

Meyer DR, Antonello A, Lindberg JV (1990) Assessment of tear drainage after canalicular obstruction using fluorescein dye disappearance. Ophthalmology 97: 1370-1374.

Norn MS (1972) Method of testing dyes for vital staining of the cornea and conjunctiva. Acta Ophthalmol. 50: 809-814.

Norn MS (1973) Fluorexon vital staining of the cornea and conjunctiva. Acta Ophthalmol. 51: 670-678.

Robert G (1920) Note sur l'emploi du blue de methylene en therapeutique oculaire. Ann d'Oculist. 157: 507-509.

Synder C, Paugh JR (1998) Rose Bengal dye concentration and volume delivered by dye-impregnated paper strips. Optometry Vision Sci. 75: 339-341.

Topical ocular anaesthetics

Bartfield JM, Holmes TJ, Baccio-Robak N (1994) A comparison of propraracine and tetracaine eye anesthetics. Acad Emerg Med. 1: 364-367.

Bryant JA (1969) Local and topical anesthetics in ophthalmology. Surv Ophthalmol. 13: 263-283.

Draeger J, Langenbucher H, Bannert C (1984) Efficacy of topical anaesthetics. Ophthalmic Res. 16: 135-138.

Jervey JW (1955) Topical anesthetics for the eye. A comparative study. Southern Med J. 48: 770-774.

Kernie MA, Proehl GA, Remington LA (1990) A comparative study of Fluorocaine and Fluress in Golmann tonometry. S J Optom. VIII: 13-15.

Lawrenson JG, Edgar DF, Tanna GK et al. (1998) Comparison of the tolerability and efficacy of unit-dose, preservative-free topical ocular anaesthetics. Ophthal Physiol Opt. 18: 393-400.

Lyle WM, Page C (1975) Possible adverse effects from local anesthetics and the treatment of these reactions. Am J Optom Physiol Opt. 52: 736-742.

Schlegel HE, Swan KC (1954) Benoxinate (Dorsacaine) for rapid corneal anesthesia. Arch Ophthalmol. 51: 663-670.

Tota G, La Marca F (1987) Ulteriori indagini su alcuni colliri a base di prossimetacaina: correlazione tra tempo di contatto corneale e l'effetto del farmaco. Ann Ottalmol Clin Oculist. 113: 805-812.

Chapters 5 and 6 - AUTONOMIC PHARMACOLOGY and the EYE. I and II

Doughty MJ (1997) Neuropharmacology of the central and autonomic nervous system, neuractive drugs and the general impact on the eye and vision. Optician (supplement) May.

Doughty MJ (1998) General Pharmacology for Primary Eye Care. Smawcastellane Information Services, Helensburgh.

Botulinum toxin and its use

Ausinich B, Rayburn LR, Munson Es et al. (1976) Ketamine and intraocular pressure in children. Anesth Analg. 55: 773-775.

Balkan RJ, Poole T (1991) A five-year analysis of Botulinum toxin type A injections: Some unusual features. Ann Ophthalmol (Chic) 23: 326-333.

Cugini U, Lanzetta P, Nadbath P et al. (1997) Sedation with ketamine during cataract surgery. J Cataract Refract Surg. 23: 784-786.

Elston JS (1985) Botulism, Botulinum toxin and strabismus. Br Orthop J. 42: 16-19.

Lymburn EG, MacEwen CJ (1994) Botulinum toxin the management of heterophoria. Br Orthop J. 51: 38-40.

Osako M, Keltner JL (1991) Botulinum A toxin (Oculinum) in ophthalmology. Surv Ophthalmol. 36: 28-46.

Powell CM, Lee JP, Elston JS (1987) Role of botulinum toxin the treatment of squint - current indications. Br Orthop J. 44: 28-33.

Chapter 7 - MYDRIATIC OPHTHALMIC SOLUTIONS and their USES

Guidelines on use of mydriatics

Alexander LJ, Scholles J (1987) Clinical and legal aspects of pupillary dilation. J Am Optom Assoc 58: 432-437.

Barrett BT, McGraw PV (1998) Clinical assessment of anterior chamber depth. Ophthal Physiol Opt 18 (suppl 2): S32-S39.

Brooks AMW, West RH, Gillies WE (1986) The risks of precipitating acute angle closure glaucoma with the clinical use of mydriatic agents. Med J Australia 145: 34-36.

Classe JG (1992) Pupillary dilation: an eye-opening problem. J Am Optom Assoc 63: 733-741.

Doughty MJ (1997) Pupillary dilation. The standard for delivery of primary eye care. Optometry Today. Nov 14 (pp. 27-31) and Dce 12 (pp. 24-28).

Hakim OJ, Orton RB, Cadera W (1990) Topical 2.5 % and 5 % phenylephrine: comparison of effects on heart rate and blood pressure. Can J Ophthalmol. 25: 336-339.

Hess RF, Harding GFA, Drasdo N (1974) Seizures induced by flickering light. Am J Optom Physiol Opt. 51: 517-529. □ □

Levine L (1985) Minimizing risks of adverse reactions to mydriatic agents in binocular indirect ophthalmoscopy. J Am Optom Assoc. 56: 542-548.

Montgomery DMI, Macewan CJ (1989) Pupil dilation with tropicamide. The effects on acuity, accommodation and refraction. Eye 3: 845-8.

Modri JA, Lyle WM, Mousa GY (1986) Does prior instillation of a topical anesthetic enhance the effect of tropicamide ?. Am J Optom Physiol Opt. 63: 290-293.

Norden LC (1978) Adverse reactions to topical ocular autonomic agents. J Am Optom Assoc. 49: 75-80.

O'Connor PS, Tredici TJ, Pickett J et al. (1988) Effects of routine pupillary dilation on functional daylight vision. Arch Ophthalmol 106: 1567-1569.

Phillips CL (1984) Dilate the pupil and see the fundus. Br Med J 288: 1779-80.

Samples JR, Meyer SM (1988) Use of ophthalmic medications in pregnant and nursing women. Am J Ophthalmol. 106: 616-623.

Siderov J, Bartlett JR, Madigan CJ (1996) Pupillary dilation: the patient's perspective. Clin Exptl Optom 79: 62-66.

Spiecker HD (1963) Untersuchungen sur Strassenverkehsstauglichkeit bei medikamentoser Mydriasis und Miosis. Der Deutsch Ophthalmol Ges 65: 353-9.

Trevino RC (1988) Pupillary dilation in clinical practice. Can J Optom 50: 167-75.

Tropicamide as mydriatic

Doughty MJ, Lyle WM (1991) Dapiprazole, an alpha adrenergic blocking drug, as an alternative miotic to pilocarpine or moxisylyte (thymoxamine) for reversing tropicamide mydriasis. Can J Optom 53: 111-117.

Doughty MJ, Lyle WM (1992) A review of the clinical pharmacokinetics of pilocarpine, moxisylyte (thymoxamine) and dapiprazole in the reversal of diagnostic pupillary dilation. Optom Vis Sci 69: 358-368.

Levine L (1983) Tropicamide-induced mydriasis in densely pigmented eyes. Am J Optom Physiol Opt. 60: 673-677.

Phenylephrine as a mydriatic

Doughty MJ, Lyle WM (1992) A review of the clinical pharmacokinetics of pilocarpine, moxisylyte (thymoxamine) and dapiprazole in the reversal of diagnostic pupillary dilation. Optom Vis Sci 69: 358-368.

Doughty MJ, Lyle W, Trevino R, Flanagan J (1988) A study of mydriasis produced by topical phenylephrine 2.5 % in young adults. Can J Optom 50: 40-60.

Gimpel G, Doughty MJ, Lyle WM (1994) Large sample study of the effects of phenylephrine 2.5 % eyedrops on the amplitude of accommodation in man. Ophthal Physiol Opt. 14: 123-128.

Tanner V, Casswell AG (1996) A comparative study of the efficacy of 2.5 % phenylephrine and 10 % phenylephrine in pre-operative mydriasis for routine cataract surgery. Eye 10: 95-98.

6-hydroxyamphetamine and other mydriatics

Huber MJE, Smith SA, Smith SE (1985) Mydriatic drugs for diabetic patients. Br J Ophthalmol. 69: 425-427.

Kergoat H, Lovasik JV, Doughty MJ (1989) A pupillographic evaluation of a phenylephrine 5 % - tropicamide 0.8 % combiantion mydriatic. J Ocular Pharmacol 5: 199-216.

Levine L (1985) Minimizing risks of adverse reactions to mydriatic agents in binocular indirect ophthalmoscopy. J Am Optom Assoc. 56: 542-548.

Levine L (1982) Mydriatic effectiveness of dilute combinations of phenylephrine and tropicamide. Am J Optom Physiol Opt. 59: 580-594.

Marron J (1940) Cycloplegia and mydriasis by use of atropine, scopolamine and homatropine-paradrine. Arch Ophthalmol. 23: 340-350.

Molinari JF (1983) A clinical comparison of mydriatics. J Am Optom Assoc. 54: 781-784.

Otsuka N, Yoshitomi T, Tusuchiya K et al. (1998) Adrenoceptors affect accommodation by modulating cholinergic activity. Jpn J Ophthalmol. 42: 66-70.

Semes LP, Bartlett JD (1982) Mydriatic effectiveness of hydroxyamphetamine. J Am Optom Assoc. 53: 899-904.

Chapter 8 - OPHTHALMIC CYCLOPLEGIC DRUGS

Guidelines on use of cycloplegics

Bannon Re (1947) The use of cycloplegics in refraction. Am J Optom Archiv Am Acad Optom. 24: 513-568.

Gray LG (1979) Avoiding adverse effects of cycloplegics in infants and children. J Am Optom Assoc. 50: 465-471.

Hermansen MC, Sullivan LS (1985) Feeding intolerance following ophthalmologic examination. Am J Dis Child 139: 367-368.

Hoefnagel D (1961) Toxic effects of atropine and homatropine eyedrops in children. New Engl J Med. 264: 168-171.

Norden LC (1978) Adverse reactions to topical ocular autonomic agents. J Am Optom Assoc. 49: 75-80.

Cyclopentolate as a cycloplegic

Dobson V, Fulton AB, Manning K et al. (1981) Cycloplegic refractions of premature infants. Am J Ophthalmol. 91: 490-495.

Egashira SM, Kish LL, Twelker JD et al. (1993) Comparison of cyclopentolate versus tropicamide cycloplegia in children. Optom Vis Sci. 70: 1019-1026.

Ingram RM, Barr A (1979) Refraction of 1-year-old children after cycloplegia with 1 % cyclopentolate: comparison with findings after atropinisation. Br J Ophthalmol. 63: 348-352.

Jones LW, Hodes DT (1991) Possible allergic reactions to cyclopentolate by cyclopentolate hydrochloride. Case reports with literature review of uses and adverse reactions. Ophthal Physiol Opt. 11: 16-21.

Rosenbaum AL, Bateman JB, Bremer DL, Liu PY (1981) Cycloplegic refraction in esotropic children. Cyclopentolate versus atropine. Ophthalmology 88: 1031-1034.

Homatropine as a cycloplegic

Fry GA (1959) The effect of homatropine upon accommodation-convergence relations. Am J Optom Physiol Opt. 36: 525-531.

Small S, Stewart-Jones JH, Turner P (1976) Influence of thymoxamine on changes in pupil diameter and accommodation produced by homatropine and ephedrine. Br J Ophthalmol. 60: 132-134.

Teitgen RE (1954) Single instillations of cycloplegic solutions. Am J Ophthalmol. 37: 940-941.

Strengler-Zuschrott E (1979) Zykloplegie mit Cyclopentolat bei Refraktionsbestimmungen im Kindesalter. Klin Monatsbl Augenhilkd. 175: 95-99.

Atropine as a cycloplegic

Ingram RM (1979) Refraction of 1-year-old children after atropine cycloplegia. Br J Ophthalmol. 63: 343-347.

Kawamoto K, Hayasaka S (1997) Cycloplegic refractions in Japanese children: a comparision between atropine and cyclopentolate. Ophthalmologia 211: 57-60.

North RV, Kelly ME (1987) A review of the uses and adverse effects of topical administration of atropine. Ophthal Physiol Opt. 7: 109-114.

Simons K, Stein L, Sener EC et al. (1997) Full-time atropine, intermittent atropine, and optical penalization and binocular outcome in treatment of strabismic amblyopia. Ophthalmology 104: 2143-2155.

Stolovitch C, Lowenstein A, Nemet P, Lazar M (1992) The use of cyclopentolate verus atropine cycloplegia in esotropic Caucasian children. Binocular Vision Quart. 7: 93-96.

Tropicamide as a cycloplegic

Egashira SM, Kish LL, Twelker JD et al. (1993) Comparison of cyclopentolate versus tropicamide cycloplegia in children. Optom Vis Sci. 70: 1019-1026.

Merrill DL, Goldberg B, Zave;; S (1960) bis-tropicamide, a new parasympatholytic. Curr Therap Res. 2: 43-50.

Chapter 9 -TOPICAL MIOTICS and their USE

Mechanisms and general use of miotics

Doughty MJ, Lyle WM (1991) Dapiprazole, an alpha adrenergic blocking drug, as an alternative miotic to pilocarpine or moxisylyte (thymoxamine) for reversing tropicamide mydriasis. Can J Optom 53: 111-117.

Doughty MJ, Lyle WM (1992) A review of the clinical pharmacokinetics of pilocarpine, moxisylyte (thymoxamine) and dapiprazole in the reversal of diagnostic pupillary dilation. Optom Vis Sci 69: 358-368.

Ellis PP (1966) Systemic effects of locally applied anticholinesterase agents. Invest Ophthalmol. 5: 146-151.

Fraushar MF, Steinberg JA (1991) Miotics and retinal detachment: Upgrading the community standard. Surv Ophthalmol. 35: 311-316.

Hogan TS, McDaniel DD, Bartlett JD et al. (1997) Dose-response study of dapiprazole HCl in the reversal of mydriasis induced by 2.5 % phenylephrine. J Ocular Pharmacol Therap. 13: 297-302.

Kay CD, Morrison JD (1988) The effects of physostigmine sulphate eyedrops on human visual function. Quart J Exptl Physiol. 73: 501-510.

Rengstorff R, Royston M (1976) Miotic drugs. A review of ocular, visual and systemic complications. Am J Optom Physiol Opt. 53: 70-80.

Zimmerman TJ, Wheeler TM (1982) Miotics. Side effects and ways to avoid them. Ophthalmology 89: 76-80.

Angle closure and its management, including supplementary use of topical and oral ocular hypotensive agents

Anderson DR, Jin JC, Wright MM (1991) The physiological characteristics of relative pupillary block. Am J Ophthalmol 111: 344-50.□□

Casey TA, Trevor-Roper PD (1963) Oral glycerol in glaucoma. Br Med J. 267: 851-852.

Clark CV, Mapstone R (1986) Diurnal variation in onset of acute closed angle glaucoma. Br Med J 292: 1106.

D'Alena P, Ferguson W (1966) Adverse effects after glycerol orally and mannitol parenterally. Arch Ophthalmol. 75: 201-203.

Friedman Z, Neumann E (1972) Comparison of prone position, dark-room and mydriatic tests for angle closure before and after peripheral iridectomy. Am J Ophthalmol. 74: 24-7.

Keller JT (1975) The risk of angle closure from the use of mydriatics. J Am Optom Assoc. 46: 19-21.

Gurwood AS, Michell M (1993) Understanding acute angle closure glaucoma. Optom Manag. May: 63-73.

McCurdy DK, Schneider B, Scheie HG (1966) Oral glycerol: The mechanism of intraocular hypotension. Am J Ophthalmol. 61: 1244-1249.

Mehra KS, Singh R (1971) Lowering of intraocular pressure by isosorbide: effects of different doses of drug. Arch Ophthalmol. 86: 623-628..

Moschini GB (1969) Azione ipotonizzante oculare dell'isosorbide. Boll Oculist. 48: 783-790.

Patel KH, Javitt JC, Tielsch JM et al. (1995) Incidence of acute angle-closure glaucoma after pharmacologic mydriasis. Am. J. Ophthalmol. 120: 709-717.

Talks SJ, Tsaloumas M, Misson GP, Gibson, JM (1993) Angle closure glaucoma and diagnostic mydriasis. Br Med J. 342: 1493-1494.

Chapter 10 - SYSTEMIC DRUG INTERACTIONS WITH THE EYELIDS and EYELID SKIN, PUPIL and CILIARY BODY, LACRIMAL SYSTEM and TEAR FILM, CONJUNCTIVA and CORNEA

Dysfunction of extraocular muscles, including eyeblinking

Austen DP, Gilmartin BA (1971) The effect of chlordiazepoxide on visual field, extraocular muscle balance, colour matching ability and hand-eye co-ordination in man. Br J Physiol Opt. 26: 161-165.

Billings CE, Demosthenes T, White TR, O'Hara DB (1991) Effects of alcohol on pilot performances in simulated flight. Aviat Space Envirn Med. 62: 233-235.

Bitsios P, Langley RW, Tavernor S et al. (1998) Comparison of the effects of moclobemide and .selegiline on tyramine-evoked mydriasis in man. Br J Clin Pharmacol. 45: 551-558.

Bittencourt PRM, Wade P, Smith AT, Richens A (1981) The relationship between peak velocity of saccadic eye movements and serum benzodiazepine concentration. Br J Clin Pharmacol. 12: 523-533.

Blom MW, Bartel PR, de Sommers K et al. (1990) The effects of alprazolam, quazepam and diazepam on saccadic eye movements, parameters of psychomotor function and the EEG. Fund Clin Pharmacol. 4: 653-661.

Casucci G, Di Costanzo A, Riva R et al. (1994) Central action of cinnarizine and flunarizine: A saccadic eye movement study. Clin Neuropharmacol. 17: 417-422.

De Kort PLM, Gielen G, Tijssen CC, Declerck AC (1989) The influence of anti-epileptic drugs on eye movements. Neuro-ophthalmol. 10: 59-68.

Donnelly M, Miller RJ (1995) Ingested alcohol and binocular rivalry. Invest Ophthalmol Vis Sci. 36: 1548-1554.

Edwards M, Koo MWL, Tse RK-K (1989) Oculogyric crisis after metoclopramide therapy. Optom Vis Sci. 66: 179-180.

Ellinwood EH, Linnoila M, Angle HV et al. (1981) Use of simple tests for impairment of complex skills by a sedative. Psychopharmacol. 73: 350-354.

Fine BJ, Kobrick JL, Lieberman HR et al. (1994) Effects of caffeine or diphenhydramine on visual vigilance. Psychopharamcol. 114: 233-238.

Flom MC, Brown B, Adams AJ, Jones RT (1977) Alcohol and marijuana effects on ocular tracking. Am J Optom Physiol Opt. 53: 764-773.

Goebel JA, Dunham DN, Rohrbaugh JW et al. (1995) Dose-related effects of alcohol on dynamic posturography and oculomotor measures. Acta Otolaryngol. Suppl. 250: 212-215.

Herishanu Y, Osimani A, Lovaoun Z (1982) Unidirectional gaze paretic nystagmus induced by phenytoin intoxication. Am J Ophthalmol. 94: 122-123.

Hogan RE, Gilmartin B (1985) The relationship between tonic vergence and oculomotor stress induced by ethanol. Ophthal Physiol Opt. 5: 43-51.

Hogan RE, Linfield PB (1983) The effects of moderate doses of ethanol on heterophoria and other aspects of binocular vision. Ophthal Physiol Opt. 3: 21-34.

Holdstock L, de Wit H (1999) Ethanol impairs saccadic and smooth pursuit eye movements without producing self-reports of sedation. Alcohol Clin Exptl Res 23: 664-672

Kobatake K, Yoshii F, Shinohara Y et al. (1983) Impairment of smooth pursuit eye movement in chronic alcoholics. Eur Neurol. 22: 392-396.

Lubeck MJ (1971) Effects of drugs on ocular muscles. Int Ophthalmol Clin 11(2): 35-61.

Mizoi Y, Ishido T, Ohga N (1965) Studies on postrotatory and optokinetic nystagmus in alcohol intoxication. J Forensic Med. 12: 19-34.

Moser A, Heide W, Kompf D (1998) The effect of oral ethanol consumption on eye movements in healthy volunteers. J Neurol. 245: 542-550.

Noachtar S, von Maydell B, Fuhry L et al. (1998) Gabapentin and carbamazepine affect eye movements and posture control differently. Epilepsy Res. 31: 47-57.

Pickwell LD, Hampshire R (1984) Convergence insufficiency in patients taking medicines. Ophthal Physiol Opt. 4: 151-154.

Sorkin L, Onofrey BE, DeWitt JD (1987) Phenothiazine-induced oculogyric crisis. J Am Optom Assoc. 58: 316-318.

Spector RH, Schnapper R (1981) Amitriptyline-induced ophthalmoplegia. Neurology (NY) 31: 1188-1190.

Tedeschi G, Casucci G, Alloca S et al. (1989) Neuroocular side effects of carbamazepine and phenobarbital in epileptic patients as measured by saccadic eye movement analysis. Epilepsia 30: 62-66.

Van Steveninck AL, Verver S, Schoemaker HC et al. (1992) Effects of temazepam on saccadic eye movements: Concentration-effect relationships in individual volunteers. Clin Pharmacol Therap. 52: 402-408.

Watten RG, Lie I (1997) The effects of alcohol on eye movements during reading. Alcohol Alcoholism 32: 275-280.

Pupil changes

Eke T, Bates AK (1997) Acute angle closure glaucoma associated with paroxetine. Br Med J. 314: 1387.

Fanciullacci M, Pietrini U, Fusco BM et al. (1988) Does anisocoria by clonidine reflect a central sympathetic dysfunction in cluster headache ?. Clin Neuropharmacol. 11: 56-62.

Freeman H (1958) Pupil dilation in normal and schizophrenic subjects following lysergic acid diethylamide ingestion. Arch Neurol Psychiat 79: 341-344.

Frucht J, Freimann I, Merin S (1984) Ocular side effects of disopyramide. Br J Ophthalmol. 68: 890-891.

Grunberger J, Linzmayer L, Fodor G et al. (1990) Static and dynamic pupillometry for determination of the course of gradual detoxification of opiate-addicted patients. Eur Arch Psychiat Clin Neurosci 240: 109-112.

Lowe RF (1966) Amitryptyline and glaucoma. Med J Australia 2: 509-510.

O'Neill W, Oroujeh AM, Merritt SL (1998) Pupil noise is a discriminator between narcoleptics and controls. IEE Trans Biomed Engn. 45: 314-322.

Ritch R, Krupin T, Henry C, Krata F (1994) Oral impiramine and acute angle closure glaucoma. Arch Ophthalmol. 112: 67-68.

Rosen NB (1986) Accidental mydriasis from scopolamine patches. J Am Optom Assoc. 57: 541-542.

Rosse RB, Johri S, Goel M et al. (1998) Pupillometric changes during gradual opiate detoxification correlate with changes in symptoms of opiate withdrawal. Clin Neuropharmacol. 21: 312-315.

Shah P, Dhurjon L, Metcalfe T, Gibson JM (1992) Acute angle closure glaucoma associated with nebulised ipratropium bromide and salbutamol. Br Med J. 304: 40-41.

Theofilopoulos N, McDade G, Szabadi E, Bradshaw CM (1995) Effects of reboxetine and desipramine on the kinetics of the pupillary light reflex. Br J Clin Pharmacol. 39: 251-255.

Tress KH, El-Sobky AA, Aherne W, Piall E (1978) Degree of tolerance and the relationship between morphine concentration and pupil diameter following intravenous heroin in man. Br J Clin Pharmacol 5: 299-303.

Trope GE, Hind VMD (1978) Closed-angle glaucoma in patient on disopyramide. Lancet i: 329.

Cycloplegia and pseudomyopia

Frucht J, Freimann I, Merin S (1984) Ocular side effects of disopyramide. Br J Ophthalmol. 68: 890-891.

Rentzhog I, Stanton SL, Cardozo L et al. (1998) Efficacy and safety of tolterodine in patients with detrusor instability: a dose-ranging study. Br J Urol. 81: 42-48.

Rosier A, Cornette L, Orban GA (1998) Scopolamine-induced impairment of delayed recognition of abstract visual shapes. Neuropsychobiol. 37: 98-103.

Thaler JS (1982) Effects of benztropine mesylate (Cogentin) on accommodation in normal volunteers. Am J Optom Physiol Opt. 56: 259-263.

Williams TD (1976) Accommodative blur in pilocarpine-treated glaucoma. J Am Optom Assoc. 47: 761-764.

Lacrimal hypo- and hyper-secretion; tear film

Bergmann MT, Newman BL, Johnson NC (1985) The effect of a diuretic (hydrochlorthiazide) on tear production in humans. Am J Ophthalmol. 99: 473-475.

Crandall DC, Leopold IH (1979) The influence of systemic drugs on tear consituents. Ophthalmology 86: 115-125.

Dollery CT, Bulpitt CJ, Daniel J, Clifton P (1977) Eye symptoms in patients taking propranolol and other hypotensive agents. Br J Clin Pharmacol. 4: 295-297.

Gurwood AS, Gurwood I, Gubman DT, Brzezicki LJ (1995) Idiosyncratic ocular symptoms associated with the estradiol transdermal estrogen replacement patch system. Optom Vis Sci. 72: 29-33.

Kofler BH, Lemp MA (1980) The effect of an antihistamine (chlorpheniramine maleate) on tear production in humans. Ann Ophthalmol (Chic) 12: 2187-219.

Mader TH, Stulting RD (1991) Keratoconjunctivitis sicca caused by diphenoxylate hydrochloride with atropine sulfate (Lomotil). Am J Ophthalmol. 111: 377-378.

Shovlin JP (1990) Systemic medications and their interaction with soft contact lenses. ICLC 17: 250-251.

Siepmann M, Barth J, Kirch W (1994) Sicca-Symptomatik unter systemischer Therapie mit b-Rezeptorenblockern. Dtsch. med. Wschr. 119: 1783-1785.

Van Agtmaal EJ, Thorig L, Van Haeringen NJ (1985) Effect of acetazolamide (Diamox) on tear secretion. Doc Ophthalmol. 5: 77-80.

Eyelid and peri-ocular skin changes

Dyster-Aas K, Hansson H, Miorner G et al. (1974) Pigment deposits in eyes and light-exposed skin during long term methacycline therapy. Acta Dermatol. 54: 209-222.

Mathalone MBR (1967) Eye and skin changes in psychiatric patients treated with chlorpromazine. Br J Ophthalmol. 51: 86-93.

Siddall JR (1966) Ocular toxic changes associated with chlorpromazine and thioridazine. Can J Ophthalmol 1: 190-198.

Westin EJ, Holdeman N, Perrigin D (1992) Bulbar conjunctival pigmentation secondary to oral tetracycline therapy. Clin Eye Vision Care 4: 19-21.

Conjunctival appearance

AL-Tweigeri T, Nabholtz J-M, Macey JR (1996) Ocular toxicity and cancer chemotherapy. Cancer 78: 1359-1373.

Arend O, Wolf S, Harris A et al. (1993) Effects of oral contraceptives on conjunctival microcirculation. Clin Hemorheol. 13: 435-445.

Boos J, Bo,elburg T, Gerding H, Jurgens H (1993) Is there a relationship between cytarabine pharmacokinetics and keratitis ?. Int J Clin Pharmacol Toxicol. 31: 593-596.

Caffery BE, Josephson JE (1988) Ocular side effects of isotretinoin therapy. J Am Optom Assoc. 59: 221-223.

Charlton JF (1996) In Eye and Skin Disease (Mannis MJ et al., eds); Lippincott-Reven, Philadelphia, pp. 651-655.

Dyster-Aas K, Hansson H, Miorner G et al. (1974) Pigment deposits in eyes and light-exposed skin during long term methacycline therapy. Acta Dermat. 54: 209-222.

Mathalone MBR (1967) Eye and skin changes in psychiatric patients treated with chlorpromazine. Br J Ophthalmol. 51: 86-93.

Skegg DCG, Doll R (1977) Frequency of eye complaints and rashes among patients receiving practolol and propranolol. Lancet 2: 475-478.

Siddall JR (1966) Ocular toxic changes associated with chlorpromazine and thioridazine. Can J Ophthalmol 1: 190-198.

Corneal appearance and curvature

Alexander LJ, Bowerman L, Thompson LR 91985) The prevalance of the ocular side effects of chlorpromazine in the Tuscaloosa Veterans Administration patient population. J Am Optom Assoc. 56: 872-876. □□

Bron AJ, McLendon BF, Camp V (1979) Epithelial deposition of gold in the cornea in patients receiving systemic therapy. Am J Ophthalmol. 88: 354-360.

Cullen AP, Chou BR (1986) Keratopathy with low dose chloroquine therapy. J Am Optom Assoc. 57: 368-372.

Easterbrook M (1990) Is corneal deposition of antimalarial any indication of retinal toxicity ?. Can J Ophthalmol. 25: 249-251.

Flemming CJ, Salisbury ELC, Kirwan P et al. (1996) Chrysiasis after low-dose gold and UV light exposure. J Am Acad Dermatol. 34: 349-351.

Hanna C, Fraunfelder FT, Sanchez J (1974) Ultrastructural study of argyrosis of the cornea and conjunctiva. Arch Ophthalmol. 92: 18-22.

Ingram DV, Jaggarao NSV, Chamberlain DA (1982) Ocular changes resulting from therapy with amiodarone. Br J Ophthalmol. 66: 676-679.

Moller HU, Thygesen K, Kruit PJ (1991) Corneal deposits associated with flecainide. Br Med J. 302: 506-507.

Oshika T, Itotagawa K, Sawa M (1991) Severe corneal edema after prolonged use of psychotropic agents. Cornea 10: 354-357.

Stern RS, Parrish JA, Fitzpatrick TB (1985) Ocular findings in patients treated with PUVA. J Invest Dermatol. 85: 269-273.

Tillmann W, Keitel L (1977) Hornhautveranderungen durch Indometacin (Amuno). Klin Monatsbl Augenhielkd. 170: 756-759.

Yasuhara T, Nishida K, Uchida K et al. (1996) Corneal endothelial changes in schizophrenic patients with long-term administration of major tranquilizers. Am J Ophthalmol. 121: 84-88.

Chapter 11 - **ARTIFICIAL TEARS and OCULAR LUBRICANTS**

Absolon MJ, Brown CA (1968) Acetylcysteine in kerato-conjunctivitis sicca. Br J Ophthalmol. 52: 310-316.

Bach FC, Adam JB, McWhirter HC et al. (1972) Ocular retention of artificial tear solutions. Ann Ophthalmol (Chic). 4: 116-119.

Bron AJ, Daubas P, Siou-Mermet R et al. (1998) Comparison of the efficacy and safety of two eye gels in the treatment of dry eyes: Lacrinorm and Viscotears. Eye 12: 839-847.

Carlfors J, Edsman K, Petersson R et al. (1998) Rheological evaluation of Gelrite© in situ gels for ophthalmic use. Eur J Pharmaceut Sci. 6: 113-119.

Doughty MJ (1990) What is really new and where do we go from here for dry and irritated eyes ?. Optom Vis Sci. 67: 567-571.

Dudinski O, Finnin BC, Reed BL (1983) Acceptability of thickened eye drops to human subjects. Curr Therap Res. 33: 322-337.

Fassihi AR, Naidoo NT (1989) Irritation associated with tear-replacement ophthalmic drops. A pharmaceutical and subjective investigation. S Afr Med J. 75: 233-235.

Fletcher EL, Brennan NA (1993) The efect of solution tonicity on the eye. Clin Exptl Optom. 76: 17-21.

Gilbard JP (1985) Topical therapy for dry eyes. Trans Ophthalmol Soc UK 104: 484-488.

Greaves JL, Wilson CG, Galloway NR et al. (1991) A comparison of the precorneal residence of an artificial tear preparation in patients with keratoconjunctivitis sicca and normal volunteer subjects using gamma syntography. Acta Ophthalmol. 69: 432-436.

Grene RB, Lankston P, Mordaund J et al. (1992) Unpreserved carboxymethylcellulose artificial tears evaluated in patients with keratoconjunctivitis sicca. Corea. 11: 294-301.

Hill Rm, Terry JE (1975) Viscosity: the "staying power" of ophthalmic solutions. J Am Optom Assoc. 46: 239-242.

LaFlammae MY, Swieca R (1988) A comparative study of two preservative-free substitutes in the management of severe dry eye. Canad J Ophthalmol. 23: 174-176.

Lemp MA, Goldberg M, Roddy MR (1975) The effect of tear substitutes on tear film break-up time. Invest Ophthalmol. 14: 255-258.

Ludwig A, Van Ooteghem M (1989) Evaluation of sodium hyaluronate as viscous vehicle for eyedrops. J Pharm Belg. 44: 391-397.

Marner K, Prause JU (1984) A comparative clinical study of tear substitutes in normal subjects and in patients with keratoconjunctivitis sicca. Acta Ophthalmol. 62: 91-95.

Marner K, Moller PM, Dillon M, Rask-Pedersen E (1996) Viscous carbomer eye drops in patients with dry eyes. Acta Ophthalmol Scand. 74: 249-252.

Nelson JD, Farris RL (1988) Sodium hyaluronate and polyvinyl alcohol artificial tear preparataions. A comparison in patients with keratoconjunctivitis sicca. Arch Ophthalmol. 106: 484-487.

Norn MS, Opauski A (1977) Effects of ophthalmic vehicles on the stability of the precorneal tear film. Acta Ophthalmol. 55: 23-34.

Raber I, Breslin CW (1978) Toleration of artificial tears - the effect of pH. Canad J Ophthalmol. 13: 247-249.

Simon Castellvi JM, Verges C, Camins JL et al. (1989) Tratamiento del sindrome de ojo seco - analisis comparativo. Arch Soc Esp Oftalmol. 56: 185-192.

Trolle-Lassen C (1958) Investigations into the sensitivity of the human eye to hypo- and hypertonic solutions as well as solutions with unphysiological hydrogen ion concentrations. Pharm Weekbl Sci. 93: 148-153.

Tickner J (1997) The treatment of dry eye syndrome by punctal occlusion. Optician 213 (no. 5605): 22-26.

Chapter 12 - **OPHTHALMIC TOPICAL DECONGESTANTS, TOPICAL ANTI-INFLAMMATORY DRUGS and ANTIH-HISTAMINES**

General guidelines on use of decongestants

Abelson MB, Butrus SI, Weston JH, Rosner B (1984) Tolerance and absence of rebound vasodilation following topical ocular decongestatnt usage. Ophthalmology 91: 1364-1367.

Gelmi C, Ceccuzzi R (1994) Mydriatic effect of ocular decongestants studied by pupillography. Ophthalmologica 208: 243-246.

Rumwelt MB (1988) Blindness from misuse of over-the-counter eye medications. Ann Ophthalmol. 20: 26-20.

Soparkar CNS, Wilhelmus KR, Koch DD et al. (1997) Acute and chronic conjunctivitis due to over-the-counter ophthalmic decongestants. Arch Ophthalmol. 115: 34-8.

Williams TL, Williams AJ, Enzenauer RW (1997) Unilateral mydriasis from topical Opcon-A and soft contact lens. Aviat Space Environm Med. 68: 1035-1037.

Direct-acting decongestants and anti-histamines

Abelson MB, Spitalny L (1998) Combined analysis of two studies using the conjunctival allergen challenge model to evaluate olopatadine hydrochloride, a new ophthalmic antiallergic agent with dual activity. Am J Ophthalmol. 125: 797-804.

Babel J (1941) L'action de la Privine <Ciba> sur l'oeil normal et pathologique. Schw Med Wochensch. 71: 561-563.

Daily RK, Daily L (1949) Use of Privine-Antistine drops in ophthalmology. Am J Ophthalmol. 32: 441-442.

Dechant KL, Goa KL (1991) Levocabastine. A review of its pharmacological properties and therapeutic potential as a topical antihistamine in allergic rhinitis and conjunctivitis. Drugs 41: 202-224.

D'Esposito M, Cortese G, Brusorio S et al. (1991) Validita terapeutica di un collirio a base di ossimetazolina cloridato 0,025 % e polivinil alcool 1,4 % somministrato due volte al gioro. Boll Oculist. 70: 303-308.

Discepola M, Deschenes J, Abelson M (1999) Comparison of the topical ocular antiallergic efficacy of emedastine 0.05 % ophthalmic solution to ketorolac 0.5 % ophthalmic solution in a clinical model of allergic conjunctivitis. Acta Ophthalmol Scand Suppl. 228: 43-6

Doughty MJ (1997) A guide to ophthalmic Pharmacy Medicines in the United Kingdom. Ophthal Physiol Opt. 17(suppl 1): S2-S8.

Duzman E, Anderson J, Vita JB et al. (1983) Topically-applied oxymetazoline. Ocular vasoconstrictive activity, pharmacokinetics and metabolism. Arch. Ophthalmol. 101: 1122-1126.

Goes F, Blockhuys S, Janssens M (1994) Levocabastine eye drops in the treatment of vernal conjunctivitis. Doc Ophthalmol. 87: 271-281.

Horak F, Berger UE, Menapace R et al. (1998) Dose-dependent protection by azelastine eye drops against pollen-induced allergic conjunctivitis. Drug Res 48(I): 379-384.

Hurwitz P, Thompson JM (1950) Uses of napahazoline (Privine) in ophthalmology. Arch Ophthalmol. 43: 712-717.

Janssens M (1992) Efficay of levocabastine in conjunctival provocation studies. Doc Ophthalmol. 82: 341-351.

Lisch K (1978) Bindehautalterationen durch Sympathomimetika. Klin Monatsbl Augenheilkd. 173: 404-406.

Miller J, Wolf EH (1975) Antazoline phosphate and naphazoline hydrochloride, singly and in combination for the treatment of allergic conjunctivitis - a controlled, double-blind clinical trial. Ann Allergy 35: 81-86.

Trew DR, Wright LA, Smith SE (1989) Otrivine-Antistine - pupil, corneal and conjunctival responses to topical administration. Eye 3: 294-297.

Wuthrich B, Gerber M (1995) Levocabastine eye drops are effective and well tolerated for the treatment of allergic conjunctivitis in children. Mediat Inflammat. 4: 516-520.

Xuan B, Chiou GCY (1997) Efficacy of oxymetazoline eye drops in non-infectious conjucntivitis, the most common cuase of acute red eyes. J Ocular Pharmacol Therap. 13: 363-367.

Yanni JM, Stephens DJ, Parnell DW et al. (1994) Preclinical efficacy of emedastine, a potent, selective histamine H_1 antagonist for topical ocular use. J Ocular Pharmacol. 10: 665-675.

Mast cell stabilisers

Alexander M (1995) Comparative therapeutic studies with Tilavist. Allergy 50(suppl 21): 23-29.

Azevedo M, Castel-Branco MG, Ferraz Oliviera J et al. (1991) Double-blind comparison of levocabastine eye drops with sodium cromoglycate and placebo in the treatment of seasonal allergic conjunctivitis. Clin Eptl Allergy 21: 689-694.

Blumenthal M, Casele T, Dockhorn R et al. (1992) Efficacy and safety of nedocromil sodium ophthalmic solution in the treatment of seasonal allergic conjunctivitis. Am J Ophthalmol. 113: 56-63.

Bononi S, Schiavone M, Bonini S et al. (1997) Efficacy of lodoxamide eyedrops on mast cells and eosinophils after allergen challenge in allergic conjunctivitis. Ophthalmology 104: 849-853.

Camarasa JG, Serra-Baldrich E, Monreal P et al. (1997) Contact Dermatitis 36: 160-161.

Doughty MJ (1996) Sodium cromoglycate ophthalmic solution as a Pharmacy Medicine for the management of mild-to-moderate, non-infectious inflammation of the conjunctiva in adults. Ophthal Physiol Opt. 16(suppl 2): S33-S38.

Hyams SW, Bialik M, Neumann E (1975) Clinical trial of topical disodium cromoglycate in vernal kerato-conjunctivitis. J Pediatr Ophthalmol. 12: 116-118.

Frostad AB, Olsen AK (1993) A comparison of topical levocabastine and sodium cromoglycate in the treatment of pollen-provoked allergic conjunctivitis. Clin Exptl Allery 23: 406-409.

Kray KT, Squire EN, Tipton WR et al. (1985) Cromolyn sodium in seasonal allergic conjunctivitis. J Allergy Clin Immunol. 76: 623-627.

Kruger CJ, Ehlers WH, Luistro AE, Donshik PC (1992) Treatment of giant papillary conjunctivitis with cromolyn sodium. CLAO J. 18: 46-48.

Moller C, Berg I-M, Berg T et al. (1994) Nedocromil sodium 2 % eye drops for twice-daily treatment of seasonal allergic conjunctivitis: a Swedish multicentre placebo-controlled study in children allergic to birch pollen. Clin Exptl Allergy 24: 884-887.

NSAID's

Laibovitz R, Koester J, Schaich L, Reaves TA (1995) Safety and efficacy of diclofenac sodium 0.1 % ophthalmic solution in acute seasonal allergic conjunctivitis. J Ocular Pharmacol Therap. 11: 361-368.

Tinkelman DG, Rupp G, Kaufman H et al. (1993) Double-masked, paired-comparison clinical study of ketorolac tromethamine 0.5 % ophthalmic solution compared with placebo eyedrops in the treatment of seasonal allergic conjunctivitis. Surv Ophthalmol. 38 (suppl): 133-140.

Oral anti-histamines

Bronsky EA, Falliers CJ, Kaiser HB et al. (1998) Effectiveness and safety of fexofenadine, a new nonsedating H1- receptor antagonist, in the treatment of fall allergies. Allergy Asthma Proc 19: 135-141.

Hesse A, Reggiardo F, Satragno L et al. (1988) Sperimenazione clinica con una nuova molecola antihisaminica nella conguintiviti allergiche. Minerva Med. 79: 883-886.

Howarth PH, Emanuel MB, Holgate ST (1984) Astemizole, a potent histamine H1 receptor antagonist; . effect on rhinoconjunctivitis. Br J Clin Pharmacol. 18: 1-6.

Katalin S, Margit V, Pisoska F et al. (1993) Cetirizine szerepe a szezonalis allergias conjunctivitis ambilans kezeleseben. Szemeszet 130: 111-13.

Leino M, Carlson C, Kikku O et al. (1992) The effect of sodium cromoglycate eyedrops compared to the effect of terfenadine on acute symptoms of seasonal allergic conjunctivitis. Acta Ophthalmol. 70: 341-345.

Nielsen L, Johnsen CR, Bindslev-Jensen C, Poulsen LK (1994) Efficacy of acrivastine in the treatment of allergic rhinitis during natural pollen exposure: onset of action. Allergy 49: 630-636.

Roman IJm Danzig MR (1993) Loratidine. Clin Rev Allery 11: 89-110.

Wong L, Hendeles L, Weinberger M (1981) Pharmacologic prophylaxis of allergic rhinitis: Relative efficacy of hydroxyzine and chlorpheniramine. J Allergy Clin Immunol. 67: 223-228.

Chapter 13 - OPHTHALMIC CORTICOSTEROID PRODUCTS and their USE

Mechansisms of action

Goppelt-Strebe M (1997) Molecular mechanisms involved in the regulation of prostaglandin biosynthesis by glucocorticosteroids. Biochem Pharmacol. 53: 1389-1395.

Madretsma GS, van Dijk APM, Tak CJAM et al. (1996) Inhibition of the production of mediators of inflammation by corticosteroids is a glucocorticoid receptor-mediated process. Mediat Inflammat. 5: 100-103.

Millichamp NJ, Dziezyk J (1991) Mediators of ocular inflammation. Prog Vet Comp Ophthalmol. 1: 41-8.

Clinical Use

Akingbehin T (1986) Corticosteroid-induced ocular hypertension. J Toxicol Cut Ocular Toxicol 5: 45-53.

Assil KK, Massry G, Lehmann R et al. (1997) Control of ocular inflammation after cataract extraction with remexolone 1 % ophthalmic suspension. J Cataract Refract Surg. 23: 750-757.

Baba S, Mishima H, Okimoto M, Miyachi Y (1983) Plasma steroid levels and clinical effects after topical appliction of betamethasone. Graefe's Arch Clin Exp Ophthalmol. 220: 209-214.

Bartlett JD, Woolley TW, Adams CM (1993) Identification of high intraocular pressure responders to topical ophthalmic corticosteroids. J Ocular Pharmacol. 9: 35-45.

Bedrossian RH, Eriksen SP (1969) The treatment of ocular inflammation with medrysone. Arch Ophthalmol. 81: 184-191.

Buckingham JC, Flower RJ (1997) Lipocortin 1 : a second messanger of glucocorticoid action in the hypothalamo-pituitary-adrenocortical axis. Molec Med Today. July, pp. 296-302.

Butcher JM, Austin M, McGailliard J, Bourke RD (1994) Bilateral cataracts and glaucoma induced by long term use of steroid eyedrops. Br Med J. 308: 43-44.

Dell SJ, Lowry GM, Northcutt JA et al. (1998) A randomized, double-masked, placebo-controlled parallel study of 0.2 % loteprednol etabonate in patients with seasonal allergic conjunctivitis. J Allergy Clin Immunol. 102: 251-255.

Doughty MJ, Lyle WM (1992) Ocular pharmacogenetics. In - Genetics for primary Eye Care Practitioners (eds. Fatt HV, Griffin JR, Lyle WM). Toronto, Butterworth-Heinemann. pp. 179-193.

Duke-Elder S (1951) The clinical value of cortisone and ACTH in ocular disease. Br J Ophthalmol. 35: 637-671.

Fairbairn WD, Thorson JC (1971) Fluorometholone. Anti-inflammatory and intraocular pressure effects. Arch Ophthalmol. 86: 138-141.

Gordon DM (1956) Prednisone and prednisolone in ocular disese. Am J Ophthalmol. 41: 593-600.

Kutscher E, Jahner H (1972) Therapie von Augenerkrankungen mit vasokonstriktorischen Corticoid-Augentropfen. Z Therap. 10: 335-338.

Kwok AKH, Lam DSC, Ng JSK et al. (1997) Ocular-hypertensive response to topical steroids in children. Ophthalmology 104: 2112-2116.

Miller D, Peczon JD, Whitworth CG (1965) Corticosteroids and functions in the anterior segment of the eye. Am J Ophthalmol. 59: 31-34.

Mindel JS, Tavitian HO, Smith H et al. (1980) Comparative ocular pressure elevation by medrysone, fluorometholone and dexamethasone phosphate. Arch Ophthalmol. 98: 1577-1578.

Novack GD, Howes J, Stephens Crockett R et al. (1998) Change in intraocular pressure during long-term use of loteprednol etabonate. J Glaucoma 7: 266-269.

Olejnik O, Weisbecker CA (1990) Ocular bioavailability of topical prednisolone preparations. Clin Therapeut. 12: 2-11.

Othenin-Girard P, Tritten J-J, Pittet N, Herbort CP (1994) Dexamethasone verus diclofenac sodium eyedrops to treat inflammation after cataract surgery. J Cataract Refract Surg. 20: 9-12.

Sousa FJ (1991) The bioavailability and therapeutic effectivenss of prednisolone acetate vs. prednisolone sodium phosphate: A 20-year review. CLAO J. 17: 282-283.

The Loteprednol Etabonate Postoperative Inflammation Study Group 2 (1998) A double-masked, placebo-controlled evaluation of 0.5 % loteprednol etabonate in the treatment of postoperative inflammation. Ophthalmology 105: 1780-1786.

Weinreb RN, Polansky JR, Kramer SG, Baxter JD (1985) Acute effects of dexamethasone on intraocular pressure in glaucoma. Invest Ophthalmol Vis Sci. 26: 170-175.

Wood TO, Waltman SR, Kaufman HE (1971) Steroid cataracts following penetrating keratoplasty. Ann Ophthalmol (Chic) 3: 496-498.

Yablonski ME, Burde RM, Kolker AE et al. (1978) Cataracts induced by topical dexamethasone in diabetics. Arch Ophthalmol. 96: 474-476.

Chapter 14 - **OPHTHALMIC ANTI-BACTERIAL DRUGS**
and their USES

General reviews

Asbell PA, Tores MA (1991) Therapeutic dilemmas in external ocular diseases. Drugs 42: 606-615.

Baum J (1995) Infections of the eye. Clin Infect Dis. 21: 479-88.

Fisch BM (1991) Clinical management of eyelid disease. Spectrum February, pp. 40-50.

Kenyon KR (1982) Descision-making in the therapy of external eye disease. Ophthalmology 89: 44-51.

McLeod SD, Kolahdouz-isfahani A, Rostamian K et al. (1996) The role of smears, cultures, and antibiotic sensitivity testing in the management of suspected infectious keratitis. Ophthalmology 103: 22-28.

Stern GA, Klintworth DW (1989) Complications of topical antimicrobial agents. Int Ophthalmol Clin. 29(3): 137-142.

Specific references on antimicrobials

Bellows JG, Farmer CJ (1948) The use of bacitracin in ocular infections. Am J Ophthalmol. 311: 1211-1216.

Besamusca FW, Bastiaensen LA (1986) Blood dyscrasias and topically applied chloramphenicol in ophthalmology. Doc Ophthalmol. 64: 87-95.

Bloom PA, Leeming JP, Power W et al. (1994) Topical ciprofloxacin in the treatment of blepharitis and blepharoconjunctivitis. Eur J Ophthalmol. 4: 6-12.

Bron AJ, Rizk SNM, Baig H et al. (1991) Ofloxacin compared with chloramphenicol in management of external ocular infection. Br J Ophthalmol. 75: 675-9.

Bryan LE, Kwan S (1983) Roles of ribosomal binding, membrane potential and electron transport in bacterial uptake of streptomycin and gentamicin. Antimicrob Agents Chemotherap. 23: 835-845.

Canzi AM, Weber P, Boussougant Y (1987) Activite de l'acide fusidique sur les bacteries anaerobes strictes. Path Biol. 35: 577-580.

Charlton JF, Dalla KP, Kniska A (1998) Storage of extemporaneously prepared ophthalmic antimicrobial solutions. Am J Health-Syst Pharm. 55: 463-466.

Diamond JP, White L, Leeming JP et al. (1995) Topical 0.3 % ciprofloxacin, norpfloxacin, and ofloxacin in treatment of bacterial keratitis: a new method for comparative evaluation of ocular drug penetration. Br J Ophthalmol. 79: 606-609.

Dirdal M (1987) Fucithalmic in acute conjunctivitis. Open, randomized comparision of fusidic acid, chrloamphenicol and framycetin eye drops. Acta Ophthalmol. 65: 129-133.

Doughty MJ (1998) Reassurance on ocular chloramphenicol. Optician. 215 (no. 5644): 15.

Dubos RJ, Hotchkiss RD, Coburn AF (1942) The effect of gramicidin on bacterial metabolism. J Biol Chem. 146: 421-426.

Dy-Liacco JU, Cruz-Nievera L-F, Thorn P (1991) A comparison of fusidic acid 1 % viscous eye drops (Fucithalmic, Leo) and neosporin eye ointment (Wellcome) in patients with external eye infections. Int J Clin Pract. 7: 81-83.

Gale E (1963) Mechanisms of antibiotic action. Pharmacol Rev. 15: 481-530.

Fiorretti GM 91989) Conjunctivitis of bacterial origin in children. Local antibiotic treatment with tobarmycin collyrium. Pediat Med Chir. 4: 421-427.

Gibson JR (1983) Trimethoprim-polymyxin B ophthalmic solution in the treatment of presumptive bacterial conjunctivitis - a multicentre trial of its efficacy verus neomycin-poylmyxin B-gramicidin and chloramphenicol ophthalmic solutions. J Antimicrob Chemotherap. 11: 217-221.

Gordon DM (1970) Gentamicin sulfate in external eye infections. Am J Ophthalmol. 69: 300-306.

Horven I (1993) Acute conjunctivitis. A comparison of fusidic acid viscous eye drops and chloramphenicol. Acta Ophthalmol. 71: 165-168.

Hunter FE & Schwartz LS (1967) Gramicidins. In - Antibiotics. Vol I (Gottlieb D, Shaw PD, eds). Springer-Verlag, New York, pp. 642-8.

Laibson P, Michaud R, Smolin G et al. (1981) A clinical comparison of tobramycin and gentamicin sulfate in the treatment of ocular infections. Am J Ophthalmol. 92: 836-841.

Laporte J-R, Vidal X, Ballarin E et al. (1998) Possible association between ocular chloramphenicol and aplastic anaemia - the absolute risk is ver low. Br J Clin Pharmacol. 46: 181-184.

Leopold IH, Nichols AC, Vogel AW (1950) Penetration of chloramphenicol U.S.P. (Chloromycetin) into the eye. Arch Ophthalmol. 44: 22-36.

Lohr JA, Austin RD, Frossman M et al. (1988) Comparison of three topical antimicrobials for acute bacterial conjunctivitis. Pediatr Infect Dis J. 7: 626-629.

Lopez SP (1954) Topical use of neomycin in ophhtalmology. Antibiot Chemotherap. 4: 1189-1195.

Mahajan VM, Angra SK (1977) In vitro activity of framycetin and gentamicin against microbes producing ocular infection. Indian J Ophthalmol. 24: 13-17.

Mayer Ll 91948) Sodium sulfacetamide in ophthalmology. Arch Ophthalmol. 39: 232-240.

McWilliam RJ, Wilson T (1951) Aureomycin borate in external ocular conditions. Br J Ophthalmol. 35: 153-9.

Miller IM, Vogel R, Cook TJ et al. (1992) Topically-administered norfloxacin compared with topically administered gentamicin for treatment of external ocular infections. Am J Ophthalmol. 113: 638-644.

Miller IM, Wittreich JM, Cook T et al. (1992) The safety and efficacy of topical ciprofloxacin compared to chloramphenicol for the treatment of ocular bacterial infections. Eye. 6: 111-114.

Moorman LT, Harber F (1955) Treatment of Pseudomonas corneal ulcers. Arch Ophthalmol. 53: 345-346.

Records RE (1976) Gentamicin in ophthalmology. Surv Ophthalmol. 21: 49-58.

Roberts W (1951) Topical use of chloramphenicol in external ocular infections. Am J Ophthalmol. 34: 1081-1088.

Quinn LH, Burnside RM (1951) Gantrisin in the treatment of conjunctivitis. Eye Ear Nose Throat Monthly 30: 81-82.

Salamon SM (1985) Tetracyclines in ophthalmology. Surv Ophthalmol. 29: 265-275.

Saraux H (1956) La collyre a la neomycine dans les conjonctivites. Sem Hosp Paris 32: 1504-1506.

Seal DV, Wright P, Ficker L et al. (1995) Placebo controlled trial of fusidic acid gel and oxytetracycline for recurrent blepharitis and rosacea. Br J Ophthalmol. ·79: 42-45.

Shen LL, Kohlbrenner WE, Weigl D, Baranowski J (1989) Mechanism of quinolone inhibition of DNA gyrase. Biochemistry 28: 2973-2978.

Storm DR, Rosenthal KS, Swanson PE (1977) Polymyxin and related peptide antibiotics. Ann Rev Biochem. 46: 723-763.

Thygeson P, Braley AE (1943) Local therapy of catarrhal conjunctivitis with sulfonamide comounds. Arch Ophthalmol. 29: 760-771.

Toscano WA, Storm DR (1982) Bacitracin. Pharmacol Therapeut. 16: 199-210.

Verbist L (1990) The antimicrobial activity of fusidic acid. J Antimicrob Chemotherap. 25 (suppl B): 1-5.

Verin MM, Sekkat A, Morax S (1972) Chloramphenicol en instillation ophthalmique et riske de sensibilisation generale. Bull Soc Ophtalmol Fr. 72: 365-70.

Weinberg ED (1967) Bacitracin, gramicidin and tyrocidine. In - Antibiotics. Vol II (Gottlieb D, Shaw PD, eds). Springer-Verlag, New York, pp. 244-7.

Chapter 15 - OTHER OCULAR ANTI-INFECTIVES
and their USE

Eyelid infections and non-bacterial causes of chronic conjunctivitis

Behrens-Baumann W, Quentin CD et al. (1988) Trimethoprim-polymyxin B sulphate ophthalmic ointment in the treatment of bacterial conjunctivitis: a double-blind study vs. chloramphenicol ophthalmic ointment. Curr Med Res Opin. 11: 227-231.

Chandler JW (1990) Ophthalmia neonatorum. Int Ophtalmol Clin 30: 36-43.

Elson WO (1945) The antibacterial and fungistatic properties of propamidine. J Infect Dis. 76: 193-197.

Fisch BM (1991) Clinical management of eyelid diseae. Spectrum. Feb, pp. 40-50.

Frucht-Perry J, Sagi E, Hemo I et al. (1993) Efficacy of doxycycline and tetracycline in ocular rosacea. Am J Ophthalmol. 116: 88-92.

Hope-Ross MW, Chell PB, Kervick GN et al. (1994) Oral tetracycline in the treatment of recurrent corneal erosions. Eye. 8: 384-388.

McWilliam RJ, Wilson T (1951) Aureomycin borate in external ocular conditions. Br J Ophthalmol. 35: 153-9.

Naggache R (1953) Topical use of terramycin ointment in trachoma. Br J Ophthalmol. 37: 106-109.

Nakagawa H (1997) Treatment of chlamydial conjunctivitis. Ophthalmologica. 211(suppl): 25-28.

Peters DH, Friedel HA, McTavish D (1992) Azithromycin: a review of its antimicrobial activity, pharmacokinetic properties and clinical efficacy. Drugs 44: 750-799.

Seal DV, Wright P, Ficker L et al. (1995) Placebo controlled trial of fusidic acid gel and oxytetracycline for recurrent blepharitis and rosacea. Br J Ophthalmol. 79: 42-45.

Valentine ECO, Edwards J (1944) Angular conjunctivitis treated with propramidine. Lancet June 10: 753-754

Van Bjisterveld OP, Buijs J (1988) Treatment of blepharitis. Acta Therapeut. 14: 371-379.

Wien R, Harrison J (1948) New antibacterial diamidines. Lancet May 8: 711-712.

Viral infections

Collum LMT, Benedict-Smith A, Hillary IB (1980) Randomized blind trial of acyclovir and idoxuridine in dendritic corneal ulceration. Br J Ophthalmol. 64: 766-769.

Liesagang TJ (1988) Ocular Herpes simplex infection: Pathogenesis and current therapy. Mayo Clin Proc. 63: 1092-1105.

Niedermeier S (1976) Behandlung rezidivierender herpetischer Hornhauterkrankungen mit Vidarabin. Klin Monatsbl. Augenheilkd. 168: 713-716.

O'Brien WJ, Segundo AP, Guy J et al. (1996) Herpetic stromal disease: Response to acyclovir / steroid therapy. Acta Ophthalmol Scand. 74: 265-270.

Pavan-Langston D, Foster CS (1977) Trifluridine and idoxuridine therapy of ocular herpes. Am J Ophthalmol. 84: 818-825.

The Herpetic Eye Disease Study Group (1997) A controlled trial of oral acyclovir for the prevention of stromal keretitis or iritis in patients with herpes simplex virus epithelial keratitis. Arch Ophthalmol. 115: 703-712.

Wagstaff AJ, Faulds D, Goa KL (1994) Aciclovir. A reappraisal of its antiviral efficacy, pharmacokinetic properties and therapeutic efficacy. Drugs 47: 153-205.

Wellings PC, Audry PN, Bours PH et al. (1972) Clinical evaluation of trifluorothymidine in the treatment of herpes simplex corneal ulcers. Am J Ophthalmol. 73: 932-937.

Fungal and protozoan infections

Ahearn DG, Gabriel MM (1987) Contact lenses, disinfectants and Acanthamoeba keratitis. Adv Appl Microbiol. 43: 35-56.

Burger RM, Franco RJ, Drlica K (1994) Killing Acanthamoebae with polyaminopropyl biguanide: Quantitation and kinetics. Antimicrob Agents Chemotherap. 38: 886-888.

Cohen T, Sauvageon-Martre H, Brossard D et al. (1996) Anmphotericin B eye drops as a lipidic emulsion. Int J Pharmaceut. 137: 249-254.

Elson WO (1945) The antibacterial and fungistatic properties of propamidine. J Infect Dis. 76: 193-197.

Hugo WB (1971) Amidines. In - Inhibition and Destruction of the Microbial Cell (Hugo WB, ed). Academic Press, New York, pp. 121-36.

Jones DB, Forster RK, Rebell G (1972) Fusarium solani keratitis treated with natamycin (pimaricin). Arch Ophthalmol. 88: 147-154.

Kurbassi M, Riazmand MB, Schuman JS (1992) Herpes zoster ophthalmicus. Surv Ophthalmol. 36: 395-410.

Liesegang TJ (1988) Ocular herpes simplex infection: Pathogenesis and current therapy. Mayo Clin Proc. 63: 1092-1105.

Lindquist TD (1998) Treatment of Acanthamoeba keratitis. Cornea 17: 11-16.

Niszl IA, Markus MB (1998) Anti-Acanthamoeba activity of contact lens solutions. Br J Ophthalmol. 82: 1033-8.

O'Day DM (1987) Selection of appropriate antifungal therapy. Cornea 6: 235-245.

Park DH, Palay DA, Daya SM et al. (1997) The role of topical corticosteroids in the management of Acanthamoeba keratitis. Cornea 16: 277-283.

Seal DV, Hay J, Kirkness Cm (1995) Chlorhexidine or polyhexamethylene biguanide for Acanthamoeba keratitis. Lancet 345: 136.

Wood TO, Williford W 91976) Treatment of keratomycosis with amphotericin B 0.15 %. Am J Ophthalmol. 81: 847-849.

Chapter 16 - OPHTHALMIC ANTI-BACTERIAL - CORTICOSTEROID COMBINATIONS

Clinical use of antibacterial-corticosteroid combinations

Aragones JV (1973) The treatment of blepharitis: A controlled double blind study of combination therapy. Ann Ophthalmol (Chic) 5: 49-52.

Carmichael TR, Gelfand Y, Welsh NH (1990) Topical steroids in the treatment of central and paracentral corneal ulcers. Br J Ophthalmol. 74: 528-531.

Donshik P, Kulvin SM, McKinley P, Skowron R (1983) Treatment of chronic Staphyloccal blepharoconjunctivitis with a new topical steroid anti-infective ophthalmic solution. Ann Ophthalmol (Chic). 15: 162-167.

Garber JM (1980) Steroid's effects on the infectious corneal ulcer. J Am Optom Assoc. 51: 477-483.

Stern GA, Buttross M (1991) Use of corticosteroids in combination with antimicrobial drugs in the treatment of infectious corneal disease. Ophthalmology 98: 847-853.

Steinbach PD, Frobose M, Sundre Raj P (1997) Fluorometholone-gentamicin eye drops vs. Fluorometholone-neomycin eye drops following cataract surgery. Clin drug Invest. 13: 242-246.

Stewart RS, Fagadau WR, Kline OR (1988) Efficacy and safety of tobramycin-dexamethasone ophthalmic suspension (Tobradex) in prevention of infection and reduction of inflammation following cataract surgery. Boll Oculist. 67: 241-252.

Surgical use of NSAID's

Flach AJ, Jaffe NS, Akers WA (1989) The effects of ketorolac tromethamine in reducing postoperative inflammation: double-mask parallel comparison with dexamethasone. Ann Ophthalmol (Chic). 21: 407-411.

Ginsburg AP, Chetham JK, Degryse Re et al. (1995) Effects of flurbiprfen and indomethacin on acute systoid macular edema after ctaract surgery: functional vision and contrast sensitivity. J Cataract Refract Surg. 21: 82-92.

Goa KL, Chrisp P (1992) Ocular diclofenac. A review of its pharmacology and clinical use in cataract surgery, and potential in other inflammatory ocular conditions. Drugs Aging 2: 473-486.

Heinrichs DA, Leith AB (1990) Effect of flurbiprofen on the maintenance of pupillary dilation during cataract surgery. Canad J Ophthalmol. 25: 239-242.

Solomon KD, Turkalj TW, Whiteside SB et al. (19970 Topical 0.05 % ketorolac vs 0.03 % flurbiprofen for inhibition of miosis during cataract surgery. Arch Ophthalmol. 115: 1119-1122.

Stark WJ, Fagadau WR, Stewart RH et al. (1986) Reduction of pupillary constriction during cataract surgery using suprofen. Arch Ophthalmol. 104: 364-366.

Chapter 17 - SYSTEMIC DRUG INTERACTIONS WITH THE POSTERIOR SEGMENT (CRYSTALLINE LENS, INTRA-OCULAR PRESSURE, VISUAL ACUITY, VISUAL FIELDS and RETINAL APPEARANCE)

Cataracts

Alexander LJ, Bowerman L, Thompson LR 91985) The prevalance of the ocular side effects of chlorpromazine in the Tuscaloosa Veterans Administration patient population. J Am Optom Assoc. 56: 872-876.

Charlton JF (1996) In Eye and Skin Disease (Mannis MJ et al., eds); Lippincott-Reven, Philadelphia, pp. 651-655.

Chylack LT, Mantell G, Wolfe KJ et al. (1993) Lovastatin and the human lens; results of a two year study. Optom Vis Sci. 70: 937-943.

Costagliola C (1989) Cataracts associated with long-term glucocorticoid cutaneous application. Br J Dermatol. 120: 472-3.

Cumming RG, Mitchell P 91997) Hormone replacement therapy, reproductive factors, and cataract. Am J Epidemiol. 145: 242-249.

Cumming RG, Mitchell P, Leeder SR (1997) Use of inhaled corticosteroids and the risk of cataracts. New Engl J Med. 337: 8-14.

Flach AJ, Dolan BJ (1993) Progression of amiodarone induced cataracts. Doc Ophthalmol. 83: 323-329.

Fournier C, Milot JA, Clermont M-J, O'Regan S (1990) The concept of corticosteroid cataractogenic factor revisited. Can J Ophthalmol. 25: 345-347.

Isaac NE, Walker AM, Jick H, Gorman M (1991) Exposure to phenothiazine drugs and risk of cataract. Arch Ophthalmol. 109: 256-260.

Koch H-R, Siedek M (1977) Linsenmyopie bei der Steroidkatarakt. Klin Monatsbl Augenhielkd. 171: 620-622.

La Manna A, Polito C, Todisco N et al. (1994) Corticosteroid therapy, cataracts, and chronic glomerulopathy: A survey on 23 patients. Ann Ophthalmol Glaucoma 26: 131-133.

Lightman JM, Townsend JC, Selvib GJ (1989) Ocular effects of second generation oral hypoglycemic agents. J Am Optom Assoc. 60: 849-853.

Lundh BL, Nilsson SEG (1990) Lens changes in matched normals and hyperlipidemic patients treated with simvastatin for 2 years. Acta Ophthalmol. 68: 658-660.

Potaznick W, Favale AF (1993) Drug-induced cataracts. Clin Eye Vis Care 5: 110-116.

Schmidt J, Schmitt C, Hockwin O et al. (1990) Ocular drug safety and HMG-CoA-reductase inhibitors. Ophthalmic Res. 26: 352-360.

Siegel D, Sperduto RD, Ferris FL (1982) Aspirin and cataracts. Ophthalmology 89: 47A-49A.

Stern RS, Parrish JA, Fitzpatrick TB (1985) Ocular findings in patients treated with PUVA. J Invest Dermatol. 85: 269-273.

Ticho U, Durst A, Licht A, Berkowitz S (1997) Steroid-induced glaucoma and cataract in renal transplant recipients. Israel J Med Sci. 13: 871-874.

Urban RC, Cotlier E (1986) Corticosteroid-induced cataracts. Surv Ophthalmol. 31: 102-110.

IOP

Akingbehin T (1986) Corticosteroid-induced ocular hypertension. J Toxicol Cut Ocular Toxicol. 5: 45-53.

Arata M, Massin M, Speir T (1978) Le timolol per os en dose unique: effet sur la tension oculaire. J Fr Ophtalmol. 1: 745-748.

Cellini M, Profazio V, Barbaresi E (1982) Comportamento dell'oftalmotono dopo somministrazone orale di antihistaminica. Ann Ottalmol Clin Oculist. 108: 901-906.

Cellini M, Baldi A, Barbaresi E, Di Giulio C (1987) Astemizolo per via orale effetti a livello oculare. Ann Ottalmol Clin Oculist. 113: 865-868.

Garbe E, Le Lorier J, Boivin J-F, Suissa S (1997) Inhaled and nasal glucocorticoids and the risks of ocular hypertension or open-angle glaucoma. J Am Med Assoc. 27: 722-727.

Gasser P, Flammer J (1990) Short- and long-term effect of nifedipine on the visual field in patients with presumed vasospasm. J Int Med Res. 18: 334-339.

Harris A, Evans DW, Cantor LB et al. (1997) Hemodynamic and visual function effects of oral nifepidipne in patients with normal-tension glaucoma. Am J Ophthalmol. 124: 296-302.

Higginbotham EJ, Kilimanjaro HA, Wilensky JT et al. (1989) The effect of caffeine on intraocular pressure in glaucoma patients. Ophthalmology 96: 624-626.

Long WF (1977) A case of elevated intraocular pressure associated with systemic corticosteroid therapy. Am J Optom Physiol Opt. 54: 248-250.

Massimilano A, Mauurizio I (1998) Increased ocular pressure in two patients with narrow-angle glaucoma treated with venlafaxine. Clin Neuropharmacol. 21: 130-131.

Opatowsky I, Feldman RM, Gross R, Feldman ST (1995) Intraocular pressure elevation associated with inhalation and nasal corticosteroids. Ophthalmology 102: 177-179.

Piltz JR, Bose S, Lanchoney D (1998) The effect of nimodipine, a centrally active calcium antagonist, on visual function and macular blood flow in patients with normal-tension glaucoma and control subjects. J Glaucoma. 7: 336-342.

Tripathi RC, Kirschner BS, Kipp M et al. (1992) Corticosteroid treatment for inflammatory bowel disease in pediatric patients increases intraocular pressure. Gastroenterol. 102: 1957-1961.

Yatsuka YI, Matsukubo S, Tsutsumi K et al. (1998) Short-term effects of nicardipine and propranolol on ocular and systemic hemodynamics in healthy Japanese subjects. J Clin Pharmacol. 38: 68-73.

Yatsuka YI, Tsutsumi K, Kotegawa T et al. (1998) Interaction between timolol eyedrops and oral nicardipine or oral diltiazem in healthy Japanese subjects. Eur J Clin Pharamcol. 54: 149-154.

Optic nerve and retina

AL-Tweigeri T, Nabholtz J-M, Macey JR (1996) Ocular toxicity and cancer chemotherapy. Cancer 78: 1359-1373.

Alexander LJ, Bowerman L, Thompson LR 91985) The prevalance of the ocular side effects of chlorpromazine in the Tuscaloosa Veterans Administration patient population. J Am Optom Assoc. 56: 872-876.

Applebaum M (1980) Drug toxicity and visual fields. J Am Optom Assoc. 51: 859-862.

Arndt CF, Derambure P, Defoort-Dhellemmes S, Hache JC (1999) Outer retinal dysfunction in patiennts treated with vigabatrin. Neurology 52: 1201-1205.

Ashford A, Donev I, Tiwari RP, Garrett TJ (1988) Reversible ocular toxicity related to tamoxifen therapy. Cancer 61: 33-35.

Aziz AA, Hutchins RK (1998) A unique presentation of chloroquine retinopathy. Ann Ophthalmol (Chic) 30: 48-49.

Bacon P, Spalton DJ, Smith SE (1988) Blindness from quinine toxicity. Br J Ophthalmol. 72: 219-224.

Bartel P, Blom M, Robinson E et al. (1990) Effects of chlorpromazine on pattern and flash ERG's and VEPs compared to oxaxepam and to placebo in normal subjects. Electroencephalog Clin Neurophysiol. 77: 330-339.

Bene C, Manzler A, Kranias G (1989) Irreversible ocular toxicity from a single "challenge" dose of deferoxamine. Clin. Nephrol. 31: 45-48.

Cases A, Kelly J, Sabater F et al. (1990) Ocular and auditory toxicity in hemodialysed patients receiving desferrioxamine. Nephron 56: 19-23.

Dulley P (1999) Ocular adverse reactions to tamoxifen - a review. Ophthal Physiol Opt 19 (suppl): S2-S9.

Easterbrook M (1984) The use of Amsler grids in early chloroquine retinopathy. Ophthalmology 91: 1368-1372.

Easterbrook M, Trope G (1989) Value of Humphrey perimetry in the detection of early chloroquine retinopathy. Lens Eye Toxicity Res. 6: 255-268.

Estrade M, Grondin P, Cluzel J et al. (1998) Effect of a cGMP-specific phosphodiesterase inhibitor on retinal function. Eur J Pharmacol. 352: 157-163.

Feiner LA, Younge BR, Kazmier FJ et al. (1987) Optic neuropathy and amiodarone therapy. Mayo Clin Proc. 62: 702-717.

Fraunfelder FT, Samples JR, Fraundfelder FW (1994) Possible optic nerve side effects associated with nonsteroidal anti-inflammatory drugs. J Toxicol Cut Ocular Toxicol. 13: 311-316.

Garcia Rodriguez LA, Mannino Sm Wallander M-A, Lindblom B (1996) A cohort study of the ocular safety of anti-ulcer drugs. Br J Clin Pharmacol. 42: 213-216.

Gardner TW, Klein R, Moss SE et al. (1995) Digoxin does not accelerate progression of diabetic retinopathy. Diabetes Care 18: 237-240.

Garrett SN, Kearney JJ, Schiffman JS (1988) Amiodarone optic neuropathy. J Clin Neuro-Ophthalmol. 8: 105-110.

Gorin MB, Day R, Costantino JP et al. (1998) Long-term tamoxifen citrate use and potential ocular toxicity. Am J Ophthalmol. 125: 493-501.

Graham CM, Blach RK (1988) Indomethacin retinopathy. Br J Ophthalmol. 72: 434-438.

Hart WM (1987) Aquired dyschromatopsias. Surv Ophthalmol. 32: 10-31.

Haustein K-O, Oltmans G, Rietbrock N, Alken RG (1982) Differences in color vision impairment caused by digoxin, digitoxin or pengitoxin. J Cardiovasc Pharmacol. 4: 536-541.

Hobley A, Lawresnon J (1991) Ocular adverse effects to the therapeutic administration of digoxin. Ophthal Physiol Opt. 11: 391-393.

Jiminez-Lucho VE, Del Busto R, Odel J (1987) Isoniazid and ethambutol as a cause of optic neuropathy. Eur J Resp Dis. 71: 42-45.

Kaiser-Kupfer MI, Lippman ME (1978) Tamoxifen retinopathy. Cancer Treatment Rep 62: 315-320.

Krauss GL, Johnson MA, Miller NR (1998) Vigabatrin-associated retinal cone system dysfunction. Neurology 50: 614-618.

Kupersmith MJ, Seiple WH, Holopigian K et al. (1992) Maculopathy caused by intra-areterially administered cisplatin and intravenously administered carmustine. Am J Ophthalmol. 113: 435-438.

Lawton AW (1984) Optic neuropathy associated with clomiphene citrate therapy. Fertil Steril 61: 390-391.

Lorenz R, Kuck H (1988) Visuelle Storungen durch Diphenylhydantoin - Klinische und electro-ophthakmologische Befunde. Klin Monatsbl Augenheilkd 192: 244-247.

Lyle WM (1974) Drugs and conditions which may affect color vision. J Am Optom Assoc. 45: 47-60.

Marcus DF, Turgeon P, Aaberg TM et al. (1985) Optic disk findings in hypervitaminosis A. Ann Ophthalmol (Chic) 17: 397-402.

Marshall BY (1967) Visual side-effects of nalidixic acid. The Practitioner 199: 222-224.

McAuliffe D, Mooney D (1978) Thioridazine retinopathy. Irish J Med Sci. 147: 255-256.

Meredith TA, Aaberg TM, Willerson WD (1978) Progressive chorioretinopathy after receiving thioridazine. Arch Ophthalmol. 96: 1172-1176.

Mortada A, Abboud I (1973) Retinal haemorrhages after prolonged use of salicylates. Br J Ophthalmol. 57: 199-201.

Nielsen NV, Syversen K (1986) Possible retinotoxic effect of carbamazepine. Acta Ophthalmol. 64: 287-290.

Percival SPB, Meanock I (1968) Chloroquine: Ophthalmological safety and clinical assessment in rheumatoid arthritis. Br Med J. 3: 579-584.

Prager T, Kellaway J, Zou Y et al. (1998) Evaluation of ocular safety: tirapazamine plus cisplatin in patients with metastatic melanomas. Anti-Cancer Drugs 9: 515-524.

Primo SA (1988) Alcohol amblyopia. J Am Optom Assoc. 59: 392-396.

Ridder WH, Tomlinson A (1992) Effect of ibuprofen on contrast sensitivity. Optom Vis Sci. 69: 652-655.

Ruether K, Pung T, Kellner U et al. (1998) Electrophysiologic evaluation of a patient with peripheral visual field contraction associated with vigabatrin. Arch Ophthalmol. 116: 817-819.

Ruiz RS, Saatci OA (1991) Chloroquine and hydrocychloroquine retinopathy: How to follow affected patients. Ann Ophthalmol (Chic) 23: 290-291.

Salmon JF, Carmichael TR, Welsh NH (1987) Use of contrast sensitivity measurement in the detection of subclinical ethambutol toxic optic neuropathy. Br J Ophthalmol. 71: 192-196.

Schonhofer PS (1997) Ocular damage associated with proton pump inhibitors. Br Med J 314: 1805.

Shurin SB, Rekate HL, Annable W (1982) Optic atrophy induced by vincristine. Pediatrics 70: 288-291.

Teus MA, Teruel JL, Pascual J, Martin-Escobar E (1991) Corticosteroid-induced toxic optic neuropathy. Am J Ophthalmol. 112: 605.

Tokumara GK (1996) New considerations in monitoring for hydroxychloroquine retinopathy. Clin Eye Vis Care 8: 99-104.

Vessey MP, Hannaford P, Mant J et al. (1998) Oral contraception and eye disease: findings in two large cohort studies. Br J Ophthalmol. 82: 538-542.

Vobig MA, Klotz T, Staak M (1999) Retinal side-effects of sildenafil. Lancet 353: 375.

Weber U, Goerz G, Michaelis L, Melnik B (1988) Retinale Funktionsstorungen unter Langzeittherapie mit dem Retinoid Etretinat. Klin Monatsbl Augenheilkd. 192: 706-711.

Wild JM, Betts TA, Shaw DE (1990) The influence of a social dose of alcohol on the central visual field. Jpn J Ophthalmol. 34: 291-297.

Woung L-C, Jou J-R, Liaw S-L (1995) Visual function in recovered ethambutol optic neuropathy. J Ocular Pharmacol Therap. 11: 411-419.

Zahn JR, Brinton GF, Norton E (1981) Ocular quinine toxicity followed by electroretinogram, electro-oculogram, and pattern visually evoked potential. Am J Optom Physiol Opt 58: 492-498.

Zrenner E (1998) Wie sund bei Einnahme von VIAGRA beobachtungen Sehstorungen - insbesondere bei Netzhautdegenerationen - zu werten ?. Klin. Monatsbl. Augenheilkd. 212: AA12-AA13.

Zucchini G, Vannozzi G, Capobianco W (1978) Sulla possibilita' di lesioni oculari da indometacina. Ann Ottalmol Clin Oculist 103: 279-286.

Chapter 18 - MEDICAL MANAGEMENT OF GLAUCOMA

Adamsons I, Clineschmidt C, Polis A et al. (1998) The efficacy and safety of dorzolamide as adjunctive therapy to timolol maleate gellan solution in patients with elevated intraocular pressure. J Glaucoma 7: 253-260.

Akingbehin T, Villada JR (1991) Metipranolol-associated granulomatous anterior uveitis. Br J Ophthalmol. 75: 519-523.

Balfour JA, Wilde MI (1997) Dorzolamide. A review of its pharmacology and therapeutic potential in the management of glaucoma and ocular hypertension. Drugs Aging 10: 384-403.

Becker B (1960) Use of methazolamide (NEPTAZANE) in the therapy of glaucoma. Am J Ophthalmol. 49: 1307-1312.

Becker B, Gage T (1960) Demecarium bromide and echiothiophate iodide in chronic glaucoma. Arch Ophthalmol. 63: 126-133.

Begg IS, Cottle RW (1988) Epidemiologic approach to open-angle glaucoma:. I. Control of intraocular pressure. Report of the Canadian ocular adverse drug reaction registry program. Can J Ophthalmol. 23: 273-278.

Berson FG (1982) Carbonic anhydrase inhibitors of the eye - a review. J Toxicol Cut Ocular Toxicol. 1: 169-179.

Camras CB, Alm A, Watson P et al. (1996) Latanoprost, a prostaglandin analog, for glaucoma therapy. Ophthalmology 103: 1916-1924.

Centofanti M, Manni GL, Napoli D, Bucci MG (1997) Comparative effects on intraocular pressure between systemic and topical carbonic anhydrase inhibitors: a clinical masked, cross-over study. Pharamcol. Res. 35: 481-485.

Crisp P, Sorkin EM (1992) Ocular carteolol. A review of its pharmacological properties and therapeutic use in glaucoma and ocular hypertension. Dugs Aging 2: 58-77.

Derick RJ, Robin AL, Walters TR et al. (1997) Bromonidine tartrate. A one month dose-response study. Ophthalmology 104: 131-136.

Derick RJ, Robin AL, Tielsch J et al. (1992) Once-daily versus twice-daily levobunolol (0.5 %) therapy. Ophthalmology 99: 424-429.

Doughty MJ (1985) Prognosis for long-term topical carbonic anhydrase inhibitors and glaucoma management. Topics Ocular Pharmacol Toxicol. 1: 41-44.

Doughty MJ, Lyle WM (1987) The development of beta-adrenergic blocking drugs for the management of primary open-angle glaucoma. Canad J Optom. 49: 195-202.

Everitt DE, Avorn J (1990) Systemic effects of medications used to treat glaucoma. Ann Internal Med. 112: 120-125.

Flach AJ (1984) Epinephrine and the therapy of the glaucomas. J Toxicol Cut Ocular Toxicol. 3: 31-51.

Fraunfelder FT, Meyer SM (1987) Systemic side efefcts from ophthalmic timolol and their prevention. J Ocular Pharmacol. 3: 177-184.

Fristrom B (1996) A 6-month, randomized, duble-masked comparison of latanoprost with timolol in patients with open angle glaucoma or ocular hypertension. Acta Ophthalmol Scand. 74: 140-144.

Gaddie IB, Bennett DW (1998) Cystoid macular edema associated with the use of latanoprost. J Am Optom Assoc. 69: 122-128.

Goldberg I, Ashburn FS, Kass MA et al. (1979) Efficacy and patient acceptance of pilocarpine gel. Am J Ophthalmol. 88: 843-846.

Gonzales-Jiminez, Leopold IH (1958) Effect of dichlorphenamide on the intraocular pressure of humans. Arch Ophthalmol. 60: 427-431.

Harris LS (1971) Dose-response analysis of echothiophate iodide. Arch Ophthalmol. 86: 502-511.

Harris LS, Gallin MA (1970) Dose-response analysis of pilocarpine-induced ocular hypotension. Arch Ophthalmol. 84: 605-608.

Harris LS, Gallin MA (1971) Effect of ocular pigmentation on hypotensive response to pilocarpine. Am J Ophthalmol. 72: 923-925.

Hoyng PFJ, Verbey NLJ (1984) Timolol vs. gluanethidine-epinephrine formulations in the treatment of glaucoma. An open clinical trial. Arch Ophthalmol. 102: 1788-1793.

Joyce PW, Mills KB (1990) Comparison of the effect of acetazolamide tablets and Sustets on diurnal intraocular pressure in patients with chronic simple glaucoma. Br J Ophthalmol. 74: 413-416.

Kass MA, Stamper RL, Becker B (1972) Madarosis in chronic epinephrine therapy. Arch Ophthalmol. 88: 429-430.

Kini MM, Dahl AA, Roberts CR et al. (1973) Echothiophate, pilocarpine and open angle glaucoma. Arch Ophthalmol. 89: 190-192.

Kruse W (1983) Metipranolol - ein neuer Betarezeptorenblocker. Klin Monatsbl Augenheilkd. 182: 582-584.

Le Jeunne CL, Hugues FC, Duier JL et al. (1989) Bronchial and cardiovascular effects of ocular topical b-antagonists in asthmatic subjects: comparison of timolol, caterolol, and metipranolol. (1989) J Clin Pharmacol. 29: 97-101.

Levobunolol Study Group (1989) Levobunolol. A four-year study of efficacy and safety in glaucoma treatment. Ophthalmology 96: 642-645.

Liesagang TJ (1985) Bulbar conjunctival follicles associated with dipivefrin therapy. Ophthalmology 92: 228-231.

Mastropasqua L, Ciancaglini M, Carpineto P et al. (1998) The effect of 1 % apraclonidine on visual field parameters in patients with glaucoma and ocular hypertension. Ann Ophthalmol (Chic). 30: 41-45.

Mills KB, Jacobs NA (1988) A single-blind randomised trial comparing adrenaline 1 % with divivalyl epinephrine (Propine) in the treatment of open-angle glaucoma and ocular hypertension. Br J Ophthalmol. 72: 465-468.

Mills KB, Wright G (1986) A blind randomised cross-over trial comparing metipranolol 0.3 % with timolol 0.25 % in open-angle glaucoma. Br J Ophthalmol. 70: 39-42.

Ngusubramanian S, Hitchings RA, Demailly P et al. (1993) Comparision of apraclonidine and timolol in chronic open-angle glaucoma. Ophthalmology 100: 1318-1323.

Pilz A (1991) Klinische Erfahrungen mit dem Epinephrin-Propharmakon Dipivefrin. Folia Ophthalmol. 16: 177-182.

Quigley HA, Pollack IP, Harbin TS 91975) Pilocarpine Ocuserts: long-term clinical trials and selected pharmacodynamics. Arch Ophthalmol. 93: 771-775.

Silver LH (1998) Clinical efficay and safety of brinzolamide (Azopt™), a new topical carbonic anhydrase inhibitor for primary open-angle glaucoma and ocular hypertension. Am J Ophthalmol. 126: 400-408.

Silverstone DE, Brint SF, Olander KW et al. (1992) Prophylactic use of apraclonidine for intraocular pressure increase after Nd:YAG capsulotomies. Am J Ophthalmol. 113: 401-405.

Sponsel WE, Harrison J, Elliott WR et al. (1997) Dorzolamide hydrochloride and visual function in normal eyes. Am J Ophthalmol. 123: 759-766.

Stewart WC (1996) Timolol hemihydrate: A new formulation of timolol for the treatment of glaucoma. J Ocular Pharmacol Therap. 12: 225-237.

Strahlman E, Tipping R, Vogel R et al. (1996) A six-week dose-response study of the ocular hypotensive effect of dorzolamide with a one-year extension. Am J Ophthalmol. 122: 183-194.

Strohmaier K, Snyder E, Adamsons I (1998) A multicenter study comparing dorzolamide and pilocarpine as adjunctive therapy to timolol: patient preference and impact on daily life. J Am Optom Assoc. 69: 441-451.

The AGIS Investigators (1998) The advanced glaucoma intervention study (AGIS): 4. Comparision of treatment outcomes within race. Ophthalmology 105: 1146-1164.

Warwar RE, Bullock JD, Ballal D (1998) Cystoid macular edema and anterior uveitis associated with latanoprost use. Ophthalmology 105: 263-268.

Watson PG (1998) Latanoprost. Two years' experience of its use in the United Kingdom. Ophthalmology 105: 82-87.

Weinreb RN, Caldwell DR, Goode SM et al. (1990) A doubel-masked three month comparison between 0.25 % betaxolol suspension and 0.5 % betaxolol ophthalmic solution. Am J Ophthalmol. 110: 189-192.

Wistrand PJ, Stjerschantz J, Olsson K (1997) The incidence and time-course of latanoprost-induced iridial pigmentation as a function of eye color. Surv Ophthalmol. 41 (S-2): S129-S138.

Zimmerman TJ, Wheeler TM (1982) Miotics. Side effects and ways to avoid them. Ophthalmology 89: 76-80.

Chapter 19 - **SOURCES OF DRUG INFORMATION AND REGULATIONS PERTAINING TO DRUG USE BY OPTOMETRISTS, ORTHOPTISTS AND OPTICIANS IN THE UNITED KINGDOM**

Edgar DF, Gilmartin B (1997) Ocular adverse reactions to systemic medication. Ophthal Physiol Opt. 17 (suppl. 2): S1-S7.

Medicine, Ethics and Practice No. 21 (1999, January) Royal Pharmaceutical Society of Great Britain.

Taylor S (1998) Optometry and the law. Part 2 - the Opticians Act. Optician 216 (no. 5665): 22-24.

GENERAL TEXT SOURCES

Crick RP, Khaw PT (1997) A Textbook of Clinical Ophthalmology. A Practical Guide to Disorders of the Eyes and Their Management. 2nd Edition. World Scientific, Singapore.

Drance SM, Neufeld AH (eds) (1984). Glaucoma: Applied Pharmacology in Medical Treatment. Grune & Stratton, New York.

Fraunfelder FT (1996) Drug-induced Ocular Side Effects and Drug Interactions. Williams & Wilkins, Baltimore. 4th Edition.

Grant WM, Schuman JS (1994) Toxiclogy of the Eye, 4th Edn. Charles C. Thomas, Springfield, IL.

Jacobiec FA (1982) Ocular Anatomy, Embryology and Teratology. Harper & Row, Philadelphia.

Kanski JJ (1995) Clinical Ophthalmology. A systematic approach. 3rd edn. Butterworth-Heinemann, Oxford

Kanski JJ, Nischal KK (1999) Ophthalmology Clinical Signs and Differential Diagnosis. Mosby, London.

Okhravi N (1997) Manual of Primary Eye Care. Butterworth-Heinemann, Oxford.

Ophthalmic Drug Facts (Bartlett JD, Fiscella RG, Ghormley NR, Jaanus SD, Rowsey JJ, Zimmerman TJ, eds). (1999). Facts and Comparisons, St. Louis, MO.

Shannon MT, Wilson BA, Stang CL (1995) Govoni & Hayes Drugs and Nursing Implications. Appleton & Lange, CT.

NEW REFERENCES / NOTES

Brand and generic name index
Incl. non-UK BRAND names

(Abbreviations 2.3)

NOTES

_____

m.j.doughty - smawcastellane information services   **September, 1999**©   INDEX